Quintessentials of Dental Practice – 15
Oral Surgery and Oral Medicine - 2

Practical Conscious Sedation

By
David Craig
Meg Skelly

Editor-in-Chief: Nairn H F Wilson
Editor Oral Surgery and Oral Medicine: John G Meechan

Quintessence Publishing Co. Ltd.

London, Berlin, Chicago, Copenhagen, Paris, Milan, Barcelona,
Istanbul, São Paulo, Tokyo, New Dehli, Moscow, Prague, Warsaw

British Library Cataloguing in Publication Data

Craig, David
    Practical conscious sedation. - (Quintessentials of dental practice series;
    Oral surgery and oral medicine ; 2)
    1. Anesthesia in dentistry 2. Conscious sedation
    I. Title II. Skelly, Meg III. Wilson, Nairn H. F.
    617.9′676

    ISBN 185097070X

ISBN 1-85097-070-X

Foreword

The ability to provide effective, safe conscious sedation is a tremendous attribute for a dental team. Patients with a real fear of dentistry and individuals with other conditions which make it extremely difficult if not impossible for them to be treated under normal conditions rightfully expect conscious sedation treatment to be available to assist them obtain the treatment they require. In addition, patients faced with the prospect of an unpleasant, possibly distressing dental procedure, such as a difficult surgical extraction, should have the option of conscious sedation to help them through the difficult phase of their treatment. As a consequence, conscious sedation is considered to be an integral element of the control of pain and anxiety in the delivery of dental care. In other words, conscious sedation is an important fundamental aspect of the modern practice of dentistry.

Practical Conscious Sedation, Volume 15 of the highly acclaimed Quintessentials of Dental Practice Series, is a succinct authoritative text on the provision of conscious edition in the primary dental care setting. As with all the books in the Quintessentials of Dental Practice Series, *Practical Conscious Sedation* presents, in a generously illustrated text, a wealth of information for all members of the dental team. For the practitioner reluctant to make conscious sedation available, this book provides the necessary knowledge, guidance and encouragement to expand their range of methods for the control of pain and anxiety. For the dental team already providing conscious sedation, this book promotes and gives lots of practical advice on good practice and the safety of patients. Although not primarily intended for students, they too can learn a great deal from this easy-to-read book.

Nairn Wilson
Editor-in-Chief

Acknowledgements

We wish to thank Andrew Dyer and Ted Dawson for their patient and meticulous preparation of the photographs for this book.

Contents

Chapter 1
Historical Development of Conscious Sedation

Aim

The aim of this chapter is to describe the historical development of conscious sedation techniques for dentistry.

Outcome

After reading this chapter you should have an understanding of the way conscious sedation techniques have evolved. You will also understand the close historical links between conscious sedation and general anaesthesia.

Introduction

The ability of twenty-first century dentists to provide comfortable treatment for their patients has its origin in the discovery and development of general anaesthetic drugs in the nineteenth century. Before the advent of these drugs, the dental patient was expected to endure considerable pain and distress. The most commonly performed surgical procedure was the extraction of teeth. Grim stoicism and occasional self-medication with alcohol were the only ways of coping.

Dentists contributed in no small measure to the early development of general anaesthesia and, later, to the introduction of local anaesthesia and conscious sedation techniques. In the USA, Horace Wells used nitrous oxide for the first time in 1844 and William Morton administered ether for dental extractions in October 1846. Both these men were dental surgeons. In England, another dentist, James Robinson, was the first to administer ether to a patient in London only two months after Morton.

Carl Koller pioneered the use of topical and injected cocaine for local anaesthesia in ophthalmology in 1884. Twenty years later, procaine was available for use in dental patients. This was superseded by lidocaine (lignocaine) in the late 1940s. Reports of dentists using nitrous oxide to provide inhalational conscious sedation, rather than general anaesthesia, started to appear

Table 1-1 Chronological development of dental conscious sedation.

Year	Developments
1940s	"Relative Analgesia" (nitrous oxide/oxygen)
1945	The Jorgensen Technique
1960s	IV methohexitone (Brietal®)
1966	IV diazepam (Valium®)
1970s	IV diazepam (Diazemuls®)
1983	IV midazolam (Hypnovel®)
1988	IV flumazenil (Anexate®)
1990s	IV propofol (Diprivan®)

in the early 1900s. By the 1930s, an intravenous barbiturate, hexobarbitone, was in use in UK dental practices for sedation.

Over the course of the second half of the twentieth century, there were further developments in the drugs and techniques used for dental conscious sedation. These are shown in Table 1-1.

Relative Analgesia

Joseph Priestley discovered oxygen in 1771 and nitrous oxide in 1772. The analgesic properties of nitrous oxide were discovered by Humphry Davy in 1798. It appears that Davy inhaled nitrous oxide in order to determine its effects, whilst suffering pain from a partially erupted wisdom tooth. He noticed that his painful pericoronitis was relieved. In 1800, Davy published a treatise on nitrous oxide in which he suggested that the gas "may probably be used with advantage during surgical operations".

No further progress was made until 1844, when Horace Wells had one of his own teeth extracted under nitrous oxide anaesthesia. Edmund Andrews, a Chicago surgeon, reasoned that the asphyxia often seen during nitrous oxide anaesthesia was due to the oxygen in nitrous oxide not being available to oxygenate the blood. In 1868 he demonstrated that a mixture of 20% oxygen and 80% nitrous oxide was satisfactory for safe and effective anaesthesia. In 1881 nitrous oxide was first used as an analgesic during childbirth in St Petersburg. In 1889 nitrous oxide was used to provide analgesia for a dental procedure in Liverpool. By current standards, the machines used to deliver nitrous oxide and oxygen were crude and the gases far from pure. Many dentists manufactured their own nitrous oxide!

During the first half of the twentieth century interest in nitrous oxide sedation came and went. Success was variable, partly as a consequence of the use of inappropriate equipment, but also because of a misunderstanding about the properties of the gas and the best way to use it. Hitherto, the main emphasis had been placed on the analgesic properties of nitrous oxide, but attempts to achieve total analgesia in every patient often led to failure. Many patients experienced nausea, vomiting and excitement-stage symptoms. Appreciation of the excellent sedative properties of nitrous oxide came later following the work of Harry Langa (USA), Ulla Holst (Denmark) and Paul Vonow (Switzerland) during the 1940s and 1950s. The change in use of nitrous oxide from analgesia to sedation led to alterations in technique, dosage and in the approach to the patient.

Langa used the term "Relative Analgesia" to describe his sedation technique. The technique involved the administration of low to moderate concentrations of nitrous oxide in oxygen (using a specially designed machine) accompanied by a steady stream of reassuring and encouraging talk. The technique, with some minor modifications, has now been in use for over fifty years.

Barbiturate-based Techniques

Barbiturates Key Dates
1912 phenobarbitone
1930s hexobarbitone and thiopentone
1940s The Jorgensen Technique
1960s IV methohexitone (Brietal®)

The Jorgensen Technique
In 1945 Niels Jorgensen used a cocktail of intravenous agents as "premedication" for patients about to undergo dental procedures under local analgesia. The method, also known as the Loma Linda technique, took advantage of the hypnotic and tranquillising effects of pentobarbitone, the analgesic

action of pethidine and the amnesic properties of hyoscine. It allowed prolonged treatment to be carried out, but the method was unsuitable for procedures lasting less than two hours. Recovery could be prolonged.

Methohexitone
Barbituric acid was first prepared in 1864 by Adolph von Baeyer – a research assistant to Kekule in Ghent. The first hypnotic barbiturate, diethylbarbituric acid (barbitone), was introduced into medicine by Fischer and von Mering in 1903. Barbitone had excellent hypnotic properties and was used for many years. Phenobarbitone (Luminal) was introduced in 1912. Hexobarbitone, thiopentone and methohexitone were classified as ultra-short-acting drugs and, therefore, the most likely to be of use for dental sedation.

In the 1930s, Stanley Drummond-Jackson, a Huddersfield dentist, used intravenous hexobarbitone (and later thiopentone) to produce "insensibility" in patients undergoing not only extractions but also more lengthy conservative procedures. He used a singledose technique which was calculated on the basis of the estimated length of the procedure. If the procedure took longer, the anaesthesia was maintained by the use of inhalational agents. The technique was satisfactory in the skilled hands of a fast worker, but there were few dentists who possessed sufficient knowledge and competence in the use of these drugs and, as a consequence, the technique did not gain popularity.

The situation did not change until the introduction of methohexitone (Brietal). In the mid-1960s Drummond-Jackson pioneered a method to produce a controlled level of unconsciousness by administering increments of the drug via an indwelling intravenous needle. Drummond-Jackson's technique became known as "ultra-light anaesthesia" or "minimal increment methohexitone". The technique was widely adopted, especially in the UK and in the USA. It was, however, a subject of controversy, and over the next two decades an increasing amount of evidence was produced in an attempt to undermine the confidence of both the dental profession and the patients. There was much discussion about whether the technique produced anaesthesia or sedation and whether protective laryngeal reflexes were dangerously compromised. There were discussions about the meaning of sedation and the definition of anaesthesia. There was polarisation of views, hostility between medical and dental anaesthetists and, finally, a lengthy and hugely expensive libel action in the UK. The outcome was a rapid decline in the use of ultra-light methohexitone in dentistry.

Benzodiazepine-based Techniques

Benzodiazepines – Key Dates
1959 chlordiazepoxide (Librium®)
1966 diazepam (Valium®)
1970s diazepam (Diazemuls®)
1983 midazolam (Hypnovel®)
1988 flumazenil (Anexate®)

Diazepam

Benzodiazepine compounds were first synthesised in 1933. Early animal tests indicated that chlordiazepoxide had interesting muscle-relaxant properties. In 1960 Randall reported that it produced "taming" of a number of species of animals in doses much lower than those producing measurable hypnosis. It was this taming effect (later observed in monkeys) which led to the clinical trials of the drug in humans for the determination of its antianxiety potential. Chlordiazepoxide (Librium®) was the first compound introduced for clinical use.

Diazepam (Valium®) was first used to provide dental sedation by Davidau in France in 1966. It rapidly became the most commonly used intravenous sedation agent for dental procedures. A single titrated dose of 10–20 mg produced approximately 30 minutes of good quality sedation, without loss of consciousness.

Although diazepam is an easy-to-use, safe and effective intravenous sedative, it has two important disadvantages. First, Valium preparations for intravenous injection contain propylene glycol as a vehicle. This proved to be an irritant to tissues and caused some degree of discomfort during injection in 75% of cases. Thrombophlebitis was also a problem. Second, diazepam has a long half-life and an active metabolite which means that recovery may not be complete for up to 72 hours.

Diazemuls

Diazemuls was introduced in the 1970s. This preparation used soya bean oil as a vehicle which was much less of an irritant to veins than propylene glycol, but the problems associated with a relatively slow recovery remained.

5

Many dentists supplemented diazepam sedation with an opioid drug. The most commonly used agent was pentazocine (Fortral®). The indications for a multidrug technique were poorly defined. Some practitioners claimed that diazepam alone did not produce sufficiently deep sedation for treatment to be carried out comfortably. In some cases, this was true, but it may also have been the result of the desire of both the patient and the dentist to produce the same level of sedation as had previously been achieved with general anaesthesia.

Midazolam

Midazolam (Hypnovel®) became available in 1983. Although it has properties very similar to diazepam, there are four principal differences that make midazolam a better agent for dental sedation:
- non-irritant solution
- a much shorter half-life
- no clinically significant active metabolites
- increased potency (approximately two to three times that of diazepam).

Despite its excellent properties, midazolam is not always the ideal intravenous drug for dental sedation. Its relatively long period of action makes it inefficient for isolated procedures of short duration, e.g. removal of a single tooth. Sometimes there are indications for the use of midazolam in combination with other drugs, e.g. opioids or ketamine (see Chapter 6).

Flumazenil

Flumazenil (Anexate®) was introduced in 1988. It is a specific benzodiazepine antagonist which reverses most of the agonistic effects of benzodiazepines. It is used electively and to manage severe benzodiazepine-induced respiratory depression.

Propofol-based Techniques

Di-isopropyl phenol (Diprivan®) was introduced in 1977. It is insoluble in water and was originally solubilised in Cremophor-EL. Following a number of anaphylactic reactions to Cremophor-EL, the vehicle was changed to soya bean oil. Owing to its very short half-life, propofol soon became the intravenous induction agent of choice for day-case general anaesthesia. It has become a very popular sedative agent which produces safe, controllable anxiolysis/sedation with rapid and clear-headed recovery.

Equipment

No account of the historical development of sedation would be complete without a mention of some of the changes in technology which have also taken place. In some cases, the availability of new or modified hardware has improved the ease of administration and the safety of conscious sedation. On other occasions, the introduction of a novel sedation agent has led to the design and manufacture of a new item of equipment. The following developments are representative:

- FailsafeRelative Analgesia machines (Fig 1-1).
- Active waste gas scavenging (Figs 1-2 and 1-3).
- Disposable indwelling needles and cannulae (Figs 1-4 and 1-5).
- Pulse oximetry (Fig 1-6).
- Automatic sphygmomanometry (Fig 1-7).
- Operator – patient-controlled infusion pumps (Fig 1-8).

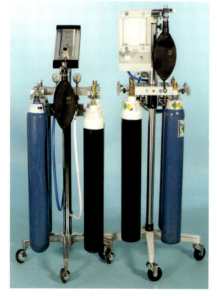

Fig 1-1 Examples of modern Relative Analgesia machines.

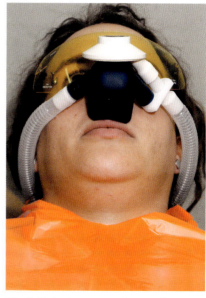

Fig 1-2 Active scavenging mask assembly.

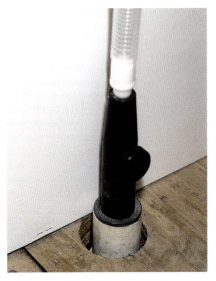

Fig 1-3 Active scavenging suction control.

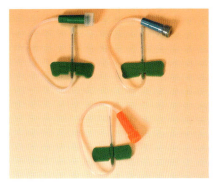

Fig 1-4 Butterfly needles.

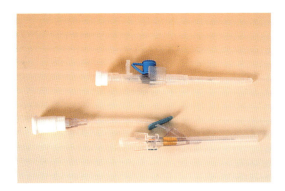

Fig 1-5 Y-Can and Venflon
type cannulae.

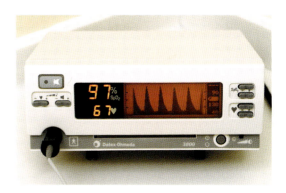

Fig 1-6 Datex Ohmeda pulse oximeter.

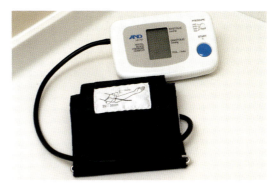

Fig 1-7 Electronic sphygmomanometer.

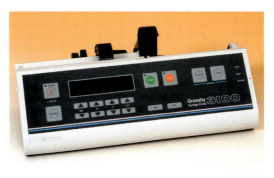

Fig 1-8 Graseby 3100 syringe pump.

Conclusions

- Conscious sedation techniques have been used in dentistry for over fifty years.
- Many techniques have evolved from general anaesthetic practice.
- The development of new drugs and equipment continues.

Further Reading

Langa H. Relative Analgesia in Dental Practice: Inhalation Analgesia and Sedation with Nitrous Oxide. Philadelphia: Saunders, 1976.

Sykes P (Ed.). Drummond-Jackson's Dental Sedation and Anaesthesia. London: Society for the Advancement of Anaesthesia in Dentistry, 1979.

Chapter 2
Basic Physiology and Anatomy:
A Whistle-stop Tour

Aim

The aim of this chapter is to outline the basic principles of physiology and anatomy which are relevant to conscious sedation.

Outcomes

After reading this chapter you should have an understanding of:
- relevant respiratory and cardiovascular physiology
- airway obstruction
- anatomy of commonly used venepuncture sites
- differences between adult and paediatric patients.

Introduction

To understand fully the principles of safe sedation practice, it is necessary to review certain aspects of physiology, in particular, those relating to the respiratory and cardiovascular systems. A knowledge of the anatomy of the upper airway assists in airway management. Familiarity with the pattern of veins in the antecubital fossa and on the dorsum of the hand is essential for the administration of intravenous sedation.

Respiratory Physiology

The major function of the respiratory system is to ensure continuous effective gas exchange so that oxygen enters the bloodstream and carbon dioxide is removed.

Mechanics, volumes, capacities and flow rates
Quiet breathing is characterised by the rhythmic expansion and relaxation of the lungs and thorax. The diaphragm is the most important muscle of respiration but the intercostal muscles contribute to the increase in the volume of the thorax during inspiration. The accessory muscles of inspiration are not used during quiet breathing. Expiration is normally a passive process

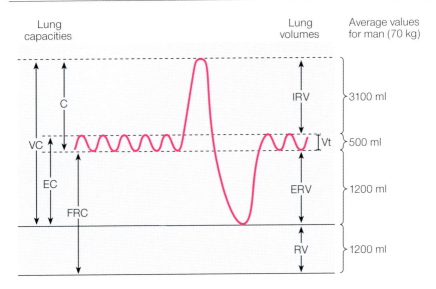

Fig 2-1 Lung volumes and capacities. VC, vital capacity; IC, inspiratory capacity; EC expiratory capacity; FRC, functional residual capacity; IRV, inspiratory reserve volume; ERV, expiratory reserve volume, RV, residual volume; Vt, tidal volume.

resulting from the elastic recoil of the lungs. Active expiration, primarily involving the muscles of the anterior abdominal wall and the intercostal muscles, is seen during exercise and hyperventilation.

The size of the thorax and lungs determines the lung capacities whilst lung volumes are determined by inspiratory and expiratory effort (Fig 2-1). Tidal volume (Vt) is the volume of gas inhaled during a normal inspiration. A fit adult patient at rest normally has a tidal volume of approximately 500 ml. The residual volume (RV) is the volume of air remaining in the lungs at the end of a maximal expiratory effort. RV increases with age and with any decrease in elastic recoil of the lungs. Vital capacity (VC) is the volume of gas entering the lungs following a maximal inspiratory effort. Functional residual capacity (FRC) is the volume of the gas remaining in the lungs at the end of a normal expiration. Functional residual capacity is important because it is a measure of oxygen reserve.

Minute volume is the product of the tidal volume and the respiratory rate. A normal adult at rest breathes approximately 12 times per minute. Thus, the minute volume for an adult is usually about 6 litres. These figures provide the sedationist with a physiological basis for estimating the initial fresh gas flow required when using inhalational sedation techniques.

The dead space volume refers to the portion of the airways which is not available for the exchange of gases. Dead space increases with age and reduction in cardiac output. The term alveolar ventilation is used to describe the volume of gas entering the alveoli each minute and taking part in gas exchange. It is important to recognise that a patient who has very shallow breathing (where the tidal volume is less than the dead space volume) is effectively not breathing at all. Hypoventilation is common following the administration of central nervous system (CNS) depressant drugs such as benzodiazepines and opioids.

Pulmonary gas exchange

Gas exchange occurs at the alveolar-capillary membrane, where only two or three cells separate alveolar gas from the bloodstream. Oxygen and carbon dioxide cross the alveolar membrane by diffusion. The rate of diffusion depends upon the:

- concentration gradient of each gas across the alveolar membrane
- area available for diffusion
- rate of removal of oxygen and carbon dioxide.

Oxygen is removed by capillary blood and its rate of transfer is also dependent upon the rate of its chemical combination with haemoglobin. The rate of diffusion of carbon dioxide from capillary blood into the alveolus is 20 times more rapid than that of oxygen in the reverse direction.

Most of the oxygen is transported to the periphery of the body in combination with haemoglobin. Only a very small amount of oxygen is transported dissolved in plasma. Normal adult haemoglobin consists of four protein chains with a haem group attached. The bonding between the chains determines the shape of the haemoglobin molecule which, in turn, influences the affinity of the haemoglobin molecule for oxygen. The affinity of haemoglobin for oxygen is also affected by other variables, e.g. body temperature and pH.

Oxygen combines loosely and reversibly with haemoglobin. Each molecule of haemoglobin can combine with four atoms of oxygen, but the association of each atom alters the affinity of the haemoglobin molecule for subsequent oxygen atoms. This results in the characteristic sigmoid shape of the

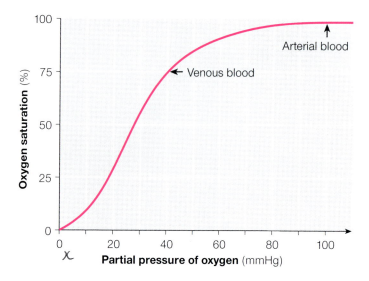

Fig 2-2 Oxygen-haemoglobin dissociation curve.

oxygen dissociation curve (Fig 2-2). The shape of the curve means that large amounts of oxygen are released to the tissues in response to relatively small falls in alveolar oxygen tension, thus maintaining optimum oxygenation of the tissues.

The oxygen dissociation curve shows the oxygen saturation of haemoglobin on the y-axis and the partial pressure of oxygen (oxygen tension) on the x-axis. The plateau at the top of the curve results from the saturation of the binding sites with oxygen. This provides a potential reserve of oxygen when the partial pressure of oxygen falls. The steep vertical section of the curve allows for optimum loading and unloading of oxygen.

During sedation a pulse oximeter is used to estimate the patient's arterial oxygen saturation (the y-axis on the oxygen dissociation curve). However, the unremitting hunger of all the cells of the body for oxygen is only satisfied by a continuous supply and adequate partial pressure of oxygen (the x-axis on the curve). The shape of the dissociation curve determines the precise relationship of the axes and thus the relationship between the displayed arterial oxygen saturation (SaO_2) and the quantity of oxygen available for cellular respiration. Careful consideration of the curve and the underlying biochemistry will demonstrate the significance of the recommendation that the SaO_2 must be maintained above 90% throughout sedation and the immediate recovery period.

Carbon dioxide is carried in the blood in solution, in the form of bicarbonate and attached to protein as carbamino compounds. Carbon dioxide is much more soluble than oxygen and so the quantity of carbon dioxide carried in solution is significant. Most of the carbon dioxide carried in the blood is present in the form of bicarbonate. Bicarbonate is formed as a result of the hydration of carbon dioxide with the production of carbonic acid which, in turn, is ionised to form a hydrogen ion and a bicarbonate ion:

$$H_2O + CO_2 \leftrightarrow H_2CO_3 \leftrightarrow H^+ + HCO_3^-$$

Control of Respiration

Respiration is an automatic process under the control of the brain's respiratory centre (Fig 2-3). The respiratory centre receives a large number of inputs, including those from the central and peripheral chemoreceptors, lung mechanoreceptors and the higher centres of the CNS. Changes in the rate and depth of breathing are produced by alterations in the firing rate in the nerves supplying the muscles of respiration.

At rest, at least 60% of the respiratory drive is derived from the central chemoreceptors in the medulla. The central chemoreceptors respond to

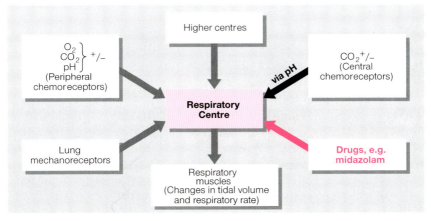

Fig 2-3 Control of respiration.

changes in the pH (H^+ ion concentration) of the cerebrospinal fluid (CSF). When the level of carbon dioxide in the blood rises, carbon dioxide diffuses into the CSF from the cerebral blood vessels, liberating H^+ ions (see above) which stimulate the chemoreceptors. Thus, the carbon dioxide level in blood regulates ventilation by its effect on the pH of the CSF. Under normal circumstances the body maintains the pH of CSF within very narrow limits.

The initial response to a rise in carbon dioxide is an increase in tidal volume followed by an increase in respiratory rate – that is, the patient first takes deeper breaths and then breathes more rapidly. Certain sedatives agents (particularly benzodiazepines and opioids) reduce the respiratory drive and cause a reduction in chemoreceptor sensitivity. They reduce the rate and depth of breathing (causing carbon dioxide levels to rise and oxygen levels to fall) and diminish the normal ventilatory response to these changes. This is why monitoring with a pulse oximeter is considered to be essential during intravenous sedation and high dosage oral sedation using benzodiazepines.

The peripheral chemoreceptors are located in the carotid body and in the aortic arch. They respond rapidly to changes in oxygen saturation (and, to a lesser extent, carbon dioxide saturation and pH), as occurs during the normal respiratory cycle.

Cardiovascular Physiology

The main purpose of the circulatory system is to deliver a continuous supply of oxygen and nutrients to the cells of the body and to remove the waste products of cellular metabolism (carbon dioxide and water). The circulatory system comprises the heart, arteries, arterioles, capillary bed and veins.
The distensible arteries convert the pulsatile flow of blood leaving the heart into a steady flow. The arterioles are the site of greatest vascular resistance. Veins act as capacitance vessels and normally contain between 60% and 70% of the circulating blood volume.

The heart receives a sympathetic and a parasympathetic nerve supply. Sympathetic stimulation increases the heart rate and also the force of contraction of the myocardial muscle. An increase in sympathetic drive is part of the body's normal response to fear and anxiety. Parasympathetic stimulation reduces the heart rate. The sympathetic nervous system is almost entirely responsible for the control of the vascular system, with the exception of the coronary, cerebral, pulmonary and renal circulations.

The average adult has a blood volume of 5–6 litres and a resting cardiac output of 5.5 l/min. Cardiac output is usually described as being the product of heart rate and stroke volume.

HEART RATE → CARDIAC OUTPUT ← STROKE VOLUME

Factors affecting heart rate

Heart rate (normally 60–80 beats per minute) is generated by the activity of the sino-atrial node; but this rate is modified by:

- autonomic tone
- higher-centre responses to pain and anxiety
- baroreceptor mechanisms
- chemoreceptor responses to hypoxia and hypercarbia
- circulating hormones, e.g. catecholamines, thyroxine

Autonomic tone depends on the balance between sympathetic and parasympathetic nervous systems. At rest, the heart beats at a rate which is mostly dependent upon vagal (parasympathetic) tone. Input from higher centres, for example in response to anxiety and pain, increases sympathetic tone and hence heart rate.

Specialised stretch receptors (baroreceptors) located in the heart and major blood vessels provide a negative feedback mechanism for the control of systemic arterial pressure. A fall in arterial blood pressure is associated with a decrease in the firing rate in the baroreceptor nerve supply. This results in a reflex increase in the heart rate and vice versa.

Heart rate is also influenced by hypoxia and hypercarbia. In normal circumstances the oxygen and carbon dioxide chemoreceptors exert little effect, but in hypoxic conditions their powerful discharge helps to maintain systemic blood pressure.

Factors affecting stroke volume

Stroke volume depends on the size of the heart, the contractility of the myocardium and on the venous return. The size of heart is dependent on blood volume and vascular capacity. In normal circumstances, blood volume is constant with the result that it is changes in vascular capacity which mainly influence the size of the heart. Venous pooling is associated with an increased volume of blood in the veins with less available for return to the heart. This reduction in venous return results in a fall in cardiac output.

The contractility of the myocardium is affected by an increase in the initial length of the cardiac muscle fibres (Starling's law) and by increasing the power of contraction of the fibres. The latter is usually the result of an increase in the activity of the sympathetic nervous system, or the level of circulating catecholamines. The normal heart never expels the whole of the end-diastolic volume. There is a small residual volume (approximately 50 ml). The amount of blood ejected in systole is called the ejection fraction (approximately 70 ml). Certain drugs, including digitalis and beta-sympathomimetic agents, increase myocardial contractility, whilst hypoxia, trauma and most anaesthetic drugs, including midazolam, decrease myocardial contractility. Venous return is influenced by a number of factors including:

- gravity (related to patient positioning)
- muscle pumps
- vascular tone
- blood volume.

Factors affecting blood pressure

The amount of blood ejected by the heart (cardiac output) balanced against the resistance to blood flow offered by the peripheral circulation (peripheral resistance) determines the pressure generated in the major blood vessels:

HEART RATE → CARDIAC OUTPUT ← STROKE VOLUME
|
BLOOD PRESSURE
|
SIZE OF BLOOD VESSELS → PERIPHERAL RESISTANCE ← BLOOD VISCOSITY

Blood vessel size relates to arteriolar tone which is controlled by the sympathetic nervous system and circulating catecholamines. Sympathetic control is regulated by the vasomotor centre which receives input from the higher centres, baroreceptors, chemoreceptors, sensory nerves and the respiratory centre. The vasomotor centre also responds directly to hypoxia and hypercarbia. Increased sympathetic activity results in vasoconstriction and decreased activity results in vasodilatation. Blood viscosity depends on body temperature, changes in the haematocrit and plasma protein concentration. In normal circumstances blood viscosity may be regarded as constant.

Airway Obstruction

Airway obstruction may occur if a patient becomes unconscious following either a gross overdosage of sedative drugs or a nonsedation-related sudden

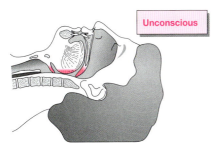

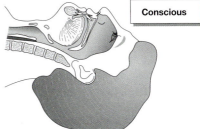

Fig 2.4 Obstructed airway.   **Fig 2-5** Patent airway

collapse. The most common cause of airway obstruction is obliteration of the oropharynx due to the relaxed tongue falling backwards (Fig 2-4). This may occur regardless of whether the patient is in a supine, lateral, or even prone position. The obstruction is caused by the loss of tone in the muscles of the tongue and the neck which fail to lift the base of the tongue away from the posterior pharyngeal wall.

Obstruction of the upper airway may be partial or complete. Partial airway obstruction is recognised by noisy air flow which is often described as either snoring or crowing depending upon the site of obstruction. Snoring suggests that the partial obstruction is hypopharyngeal; crowing suggests laryngospasm. Snoring is not uncommon in patients being treated under conscious sedation. Complete airway obstruction is indicated by the absence of air movement at the mouth and is silent. Although this may be confused with apnoea, inspection of the chest for movement (or attempts at movement) will usually clarify the diagnosis.

The initial – and the most important – step in managing airway obstruction involves opening the airway by head tilt; that is, extending the head at the atlanto-occipital joint (Fig 2-5). However, this may not, in itself, be sufficient to ensure a patent airway and additional measures are frequently necessary. These include chin lift, neck lift, or the "triple airway manoeuvre". This involves displacement of the mandible anteriorly, by lifting at the angles, whilst maintaining both head tilt and a slightly opened mouth. It is necessary to keep the jaws slightly apart in a significant proportion of unconscious patients as expiratory nasopharyngeal obstruction may occur when the mouth is closed. Oral (Guedel) airways lift the tongue away from the posterior pharyngeal wall and also keep the jaws slightly apart (Fig 2-6).

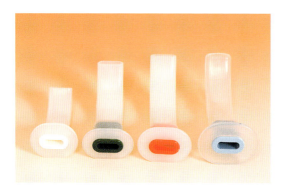

Fig 2-6 Guedel oral airways (sizes 1-4).

Airway obstruction occurring during sedation MUST be managed promptly and effectively. All treatment must cease whilst the above measures are being instigated. Ineffective management of serious airway obstruction causes hypoxia and hypercarbia which, if uncorrected, may lead to cardiorespiratory arrest.

Superficial Veins of the Forearm and the Dorsum of the Hand

Successful intravenous cannulation calls for an accessible vein. The dorsum of the hand and the flexor surface of the forearm generally provide a choice of suitable veins but other sites may need to be considered, in particular, in those individuals who have received numerous intravenous injections from healthcare professionals or by themselves. The pattern of veins varies enormously so the following diagrams and notes must be interpreted with caution. Venepuncture cannot be learned from a book, but a little anatomical knowledge will greatly increase the chances of success.

There is no single best site for venepuncture. Sedationists should avoid falling into the trap of using the same area (dorsum of hand or antecubital fossa) on every patient. The ideal vein for venepuncture is one which is of medium size (very large veins are sometimes difficult to enter with a small cannula), visible and reasonably well tethered to the underlying tissues. It is sensible to survey both the dorsum of the hand (Fig 2-7) and the antecubital fossa (Fig 2-8) on both arms before making a final decision. Some patients express a preference but, unfortunately, this is not always for the most accessible vein. Other patients appear to enjoy the challenge offered by their "difficult" veins. Intravenous drug users are often particularly difficult to cannulate and it is sometimes better to let them have a go, but be prepared for some unusual approaches.

Veins of the hand

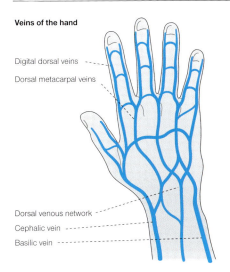

Digital dorsal veins

Dorsal metacarpal veins

Dorsal venous network

Cephalic vein

Basilic vein

Fig 2-7 Dorsal hand veins.

Veins of the forearm

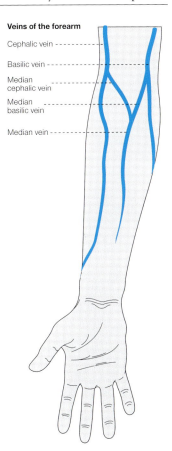

Cephalic vein

Basilic vein

Median
cephalic vein

Median
basilic vein

Median vein

Fig 2-8 Forearm and antecubital fossa veins.

In the antecubital fossa, the large median basilic vein is a tempting target, but it is often quite mobile and easily slips away from the tip of the cannula. Stabilisation of the vein may flatten it and make a clean entry into the lumen difficult. This vein overlies the brachial artery and the median nerve, either of which may be entered or damaged if the angle of approach is too steep and the cannula penetrates too deeply. The median cephalic vein is usually smaller, but is less mobile and does not overlie any important structures. The cephalic vein is often visible and is another safe choice.

There are few hazards associated with the dorsum of the hand, but the veins are sometimes quite small and tortuous. There is often marked variation between the veins of the left and right hands. It is probably sensible to avoid

21

using these veins in patients whose professional activity might be affected by a failed venepuncture and the resulting haematoma. Concert pianists, television presenters and even dentists come to mind!

The veins on the flexor surface of the wrist are sometimes useful when other sites have proved difficult or impossible. These veins are usually very narrow but reasonably well tethered and so venepuncture (using a very small-gauge cannula or even a butterfly needle) is often relatively straightforward. Contrary to popular belief, venepuncture at this site is no more (or less) uncomfortable than at other, more conventional, sites.

The great (long) saphenous vein, as it passes in front of the medial malleolus, may also be considered, although patients may be surprised when asked to remove their shoe and sock in preparation for dental treatment.

Some Differences Between Adults and Children

Children, in particular very young ones, should not be thought of as small adults. There are a number of important anatomical and physiological differences between the child and the adult patient which are relevant to the use of sedation for paediatric dental patients.

Metabolism: Children have a higher metabolic rate than adults. This leads to increased oxygen consumption and increased carbon dioxide production. The younger the child, the higher is the metabolic rate.

Airway: The head and tongue are relatively large. The neck is shorter and the larynx located higher and more anteriorly. The trachea is proportionately narrower compared with adults. Children tend to breathe through the mouth rather than through the nose.

Respiration: Tidal volume is usually smaller than in adults, but the respiratory rate is increased. The respiratory rate for young children is normally between 15 and 20 breaths per minute. This means that the minute volume (the product of the tidal volume and the respiratory rate) of children and adults is much more similar than might be expected from a simple comparison of size. An initial fresh gas flow rate of 6 l/min is therefore a reasonable starting point for the administration of inhalational sedation for both adults and children (see Chapter 6). The inspiratory phase of breathing tends to be more diaphragmatic as the ribs are horizontal, reducing the lateral expansion of the chest.

Circulation: Children between 5 and 12 years of age have a higher heart rate (80–120 beats per minute) than adults although arterial blood pressure is lower (typically 90–110 mmHg, systolic). Haemoglobin levels are increased. The superficial veins are smaller than in adults and may have more fatty tissue covering them. This may make venepuncture difficult. The brachial pulse is often more easily palpated than the radial or even the carotid pulse. Arterial oxygen saturation measurements and pulse oximeter alarm limits are similar for adults and children.

Conclusions

- A knowledge of basic cardiorespiratory physiology is important for practising safe, effective conscious sedation.
- Efficient airway management and cannulation depend on a sound knowledge of the relevant anatomy.
- Children should not be regarded as small adults.

Further Reading

Adams AP, Cashman JN. Anaesthesia, Analgesia and Intensive Care. London: Edward Arnold, 1991.

Last RJ. Superficial veins of the forearm: the surgical anatomy in relation to intravenous injection. In: Sykes P (Ed.). Drummond-Jackson's Dental Sedation and Anaesthesia. London: Society for the Advancement of Anaesthesia in Dentistry, 1979.

Chapter 3
Pharmacology

Aim

The aim of this chapter is to describe the pharmacology of the drugs used for conscious sedation, with emphasis on their clinical effects.

Outcome

After reading this chapter you should have a basic understanding of the pharmacology of inhalational, intravenous and oral drugs used in conscious sedation.

Introduction

The safe administration of any drug requires a knowledge of its pharmacology, which is classically considered under the headings of pharmacokinetics and pharmacodynamics. These subjects are potentially highly complicated and confusing to the non-expert. Fortunately, dental sedationists need only a basic working knowledge of sedative agents and the drugs with which the agents may interact (Table 3-1).

The drugs most commonly used for dental sedation are the benzodiazepines for intravenous sedation and nitrous oxide and oxygen for inhalational sedation. These will be described in detail. Reference, however, will also be made to other agents and routes of administration which are being used and/or investigated for use in dentistry, including propofol and transmucosal benzodiazepines.

Routes of Administration

Drugs which produce conscious sedation and analgesia may be administered by a variety of methods. The choice of route depends on the drug itself, how quickly a response is required, and whether the effect is required locally or systemically. The various routes are:

Table 3-1 Useful definitions.

Term	Definition
pharmacokinetics	description of drug absorption, distribution, redistribution, metabolism and excretion. *How the body affects drugs*
pharmacodynamics	description of the effects of drugs. *How drugs affect the body*
active metabolites	products of drug breakdown which have pharmacological effects of their own, usually similar in nature to that of the parent drug
cumulative effects	certain drugs are short-acting because of redistribution within the body – if repeated doses are given they accumulate in the body and their duration of action increases
half-life	time for the plasma concentration of a drug to fall to half its original value. Complete elimination involves removal of the drug from the receptor sites (sometimes called the redistribution half-life or alpha-phase) and then metabolism and excretion (the elimination half-life or beta-phase). Redistribution time is usually shorter than elimination time
first-pass metabolism	the portion of a dose of drug which is broken down by the liver on first passage through the portal circulation (applies only to orally administered drugs)
lipid solubility	the affinity of a drug for lipids. As biological membranes are mostly lipid in composition, lipid-soluble drugs reach the site of action quickly
minimum alveolar concentration (MAC)	the alveolar concentration of an inhalation agent which will prevent movement to a reproducible surgical stimulus in 50% of subjects (= potency). High value = low potency
blood gas solubility	determines the rate at which the concentration of gas in the CNS equilibrates with that being inhaled (= the speed of induction and recovery). Low value = rapid effects
recovery	in the context of dental sedation this refers to the recovery of the motor and mental functions impaired by sedation. This means regaining the ability to stand and walk unaided, coordinate fine movements and judge distance and time correctly
therapeutic index	the ratio between the dose of a drug which produces unwanted effects and the dose which produces therapeutic effects. A safe drug has a high therapeutic index

- inhalational
- intravenous
- oral
- sublingual
- intranasal
- intramuscular
- rectal.

Drugs administered by inhalation are absorbed by the pulmonary circulation. Parenteral (by injection) administration is, by contrast, much faster acting – emergency drugs are almost all given by this route. Oral administration may be more pleasant for a needle-phobic patient, but absorption is unpredictable and time-consuming because the rate of gastric emptying is altered by anxiety, disease, other drugs and the presence of food. Oral drugs are also subject to first-pass metabolism.

It is important to remember that whatever the route of administration, all sedative drugs travel to their target sites via the systemic circulation.

Pharmacokinetics

A consideration of the pharmacokinetics and pharmacodynamics of available sedative drugs is important when choosing the most appropriate agent for each individual patient. The degree of protein binding of a drug alters its availability. A portion of the drug administered is dissolved in plasma (the active form) whilst the rest is bound to plasma proteins and is not free to combine with receptor sites. Some disease processes change the proportion of bound drug. Similarly, two drugs can compete for the same binding site and thereby increase the free concentration of one or both agents. Either of these mechanisms may alter the expected clinical effects.
Drugs are eliminated by a variety of routes. Most of the inhalational agents used for sedation are excreted through the lungs. For benzodiazepines, the most important organs are the liver and the kidneys which metabolise and excrete these drugs. The measure of elimination of a drug is the half-life (see Table 3-1).

The properties and route of administration of different drugs determine the speed of absorption and distribution and hence the speed of onset of the sedative effect. A drug with rapid metabolism and excretion produces a swift recovery and earlier discharge for the patient.

Pharmacodynamics

Pharmacodynamics describes the effect the drug has on the patient and includes both desirable and undesirable effects. The definitions of both types of effect are not fixed, but depend upon individual circumstances and what one is trying to achieve. For example, midazolam can produce unconsciousness. In the case of conscious sedation, this pharmacodynamic property is clearly undesirable and potentially harmful. In contrast, an anaesthetist might choose midazolam to induce anaesthesia slowly and gently for a patient who has severe cardiac disease to avoid the cardiodepressant actions of other induction agents.

Most sedative drugs elicit a response via receptors which are specific to each drug. Receptors are located in cell membranes. When drugs bind to receptors in the CNS these are altered and the activity of the cell is either stimulated or inhibited. These drugs are called agonists. Midazolam is a benzodiazepine agonist. Drugs which act to displace agonists from the receptor sites thus terminating their effects are known as antagonists. Flumazenil is a benzodiazepine antagonist. A drug which binds to the receptor site to produce the opposite effect to an agonist is known as an inverse agonist. An example would be a drug which acts at benzodiazepine receptors to induce anxiety and alertness. However, it is doubtful that there would be much of a market for such an agent.

Properties of the Ideal Sedative Drug

- Comfortable, non-threatening method of administration
- rapid onset
- predictable sedative/anxiolytic action
- controllable duration of action
- produces analgesia
- no side effects
- rapid and complete recovery.

Intravenous Agents

Properties of an Ideal Intravenous Sedation Agent

Injection characteristics	Painless
Anxiolysis	Yes
Analgesia	Yes
Cardiorespiratory stability	Stable
Ease of titration	Easy
Induction and recovery rate	Rapid
Metabolism	0%
Potency	Weak
Speed of change in sedation level	Rapid
Reversibility	Yes
Systemic toxicity	None
Storage/shelf-life	Stable/long

The benzodiazepines

The first clinically useful benzodiazepine, chlordiazepoxide (Librium®) was synthesised in the late 1950s by F Hoffman-La Roche & Co Ltd (Fig 3-1). All benzodiazepines have a common core structure with individual differences which determine their solubility and precise actions (Fig 3-2). Diazepam (Valium®) was introduced in clinical practice in 1963 and was first used for dental sedation in 1966 (Fig 3-3). Midazolam (Hypnovel®) became available in 1983 (Fig 3-4). Its advantages over diazepam soon made it the drug of choice for intravenous sedation for dentistry. Other benzodiazepines – for example, temazepam and lorazepam, have also been used to produce conscious sedation.

The benzodiazepine group of drugs has a number of desirable pharmacodynamic properties which make these agents useful for conscious sedation.

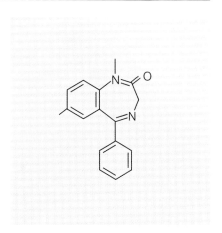

Fig 3-1 Chlordiazepoxide.

Fig 3-2 Core benzodiazepine molecule.

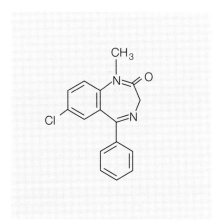

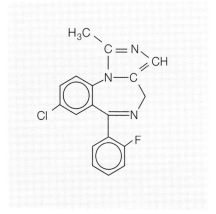

Fig 3-3 Diazepam.

Fig 3-4 Midazolam.

These include:
- anxiolysis
- sedation
- muscle relaxation
- anterograde amnesia.

Another desirable therapeutic property of benzodiazepines is their anticonvulsant action.

30

For the sedationist, the most significant *undesirable* property of these drugs is respiratory depression, which, is usually easily managed but requires careful monitoring. Benzodiazepines have the potential to produce dependency as a result of long-term use or abuse. This is not a problem when midazolam is used for conscious sedation.

Diazepam

Diazepam produces excellent sedation and was for many years the drug of choice for dental sedation. However, it has a number of disadvantages which have resulted in its being superseded by midazolam. Diazepam is insoluble in water and the first commercially available preparation, Valium®, was made soluble by mixing it with the organic solvents propylene glycol, ethyl alcohol and sodium benzoate in benzoic acid. Intravenous administration of Valium® was frequently painful due to the presence of these solvents which sometimes also caused thrombophlebitis. An alternative preparation, Diazemuls® contains an oil-in-water emulsion, is non-irritant and does not damage veins.

Many practitioners considered that diazepam on its own was not sufficiently potent for extremely anxious patients or for those undergoing surgical procedures which led to the practice of adding an opioid to enhance the sedative effect. The most commonly used drug was pentazocine, marketed as Fortral®. This technique should now be regarded as of historical interest only since adequate sedation is usually easily achieved with midazolam alone. Midazolam is at least twice as potent a sedative as diazepam on a weight for weight basis.

Midazolam

Midazolam (Hypnovel®) is currently available as two injectable preparations in 2 ml and 5 ml ampoules, each of which contains 10 mg of the drug (Fig 3-5). It is stable in aqueous solution and is non-irritant on injection. The advantage of using the 10 mg in 5 ml preparation is that it is easier to administer by titration. Titration means administering the drug slowly in small volume increments whilst assessing the patient's response. This mode of administration ensures that patients receive an adequate but not excessive dose of the sedative agent. It is absolutely impossible to predict the correct sedative dose of intravenous midazolam for any individual patient on the basis of their weight, height, Body Mass Index (BMI) or the apparent degree of anxiety.

Midazolam: Properties	
Water soluble	Yes
Solvent	Aqueous
Irritant	No
Presentation	10 mg/5 ml or 10 mg/2 ml
Distribution half-life	6–15 mins
Elimination half-life	1.5–2 hours
Usual dose	2–7.5 mg
Late active metabolites	None
Analgesia	No

In the UK midazolam is only available in a form suitable for parenteral administration. However, this formulation has been successfully mixed with other liquids (for example, fruit juices) for oral use. Similarly, the 10 mg in 2 ml formulation has been used as an intranasal spray. These methods of administration have proved useful for those patients who refuse or cannot be given intravenous injections.

Temazepam

Temazepam is no longer considered to be the drug of choice as an oral alternative to intravenous or inhalational sedation in the dental surgery. It may, however, have a place in the management of pre-appointment anxiety. For example, temazepam may be prescribed to ensure a satisfactory night's sleep prior to a dental visit.

Temazepam is a minor metabolite of diazepam which is impossible to solubilise and is therefore not available in an injectable form. It has been produced in various forms: tablet, gel-filled capsule and an elixir for oral administration (Fig 3-6). However, the capsule formulation has now been withdrawn due to inappropriate intravenous use by recreational drug users.

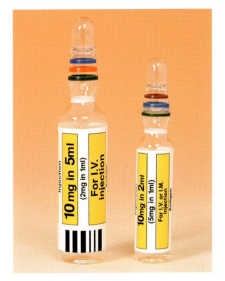

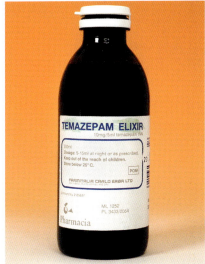

Fig 3-5 Midazolam ampoules (10 mg/5 ml and 10 mg/2 ml).

Fig 3-6 Temazepam elixir (10 mg/5 ml).

As a result of this misuse it is now categorised as a UK Schedule 3 Controlled Drug.

The different formulations have different rates of absorption, but temazepam is reasonably rapidly absorbed following oral administration. The sedative effects are usually clinically apparent for at least 45 minutes. Temazepam has a relatively short elimination half-life (5–11 hours) which makes it a useful drug for conscious sedation.

Flumazenil

Flumazenil (Anexate®) is a specific benzodiazepine antagonist (Fig 3-7). It has the same core structure as all other benzodiazepines (Fig 3-8). However, as it has a stronger affinity for the receptors than most agonists, including midazolam, it will displace them. Flumazenil reverses the anxiolytic, sedative and respiratory depressant effects of midazolam but has no clinically apparent sedative or stimulant effects. It does not reverse the anterograde amnesia induced by midazolam. Therefore, the loss of memory of unpleasant events which took place before reversal with flumazenil is retained. Flumazenil is useful for both elective and emergency reversal of sedation.

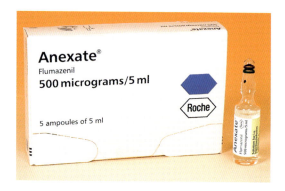

Fig 3-7 Flumazenil ampoule (500 micrograms/5 ml)

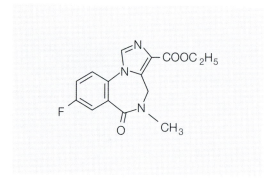

Fig 3-8 Flumazenil.

Flumazenil has a shorter half-life than midazolam. When it was first introduced, in 1988, there was a suggestion that administering flumazenil to a sedated patient would result in a short period of reversal followed by "resedation" some 50–60 minutes after the flumazenil was given. This is not true. The displaced midazolam continues to be redistributed and metabolised independently of the presence of flumazenil. The cessation of action of flumazenil (approximately 50 minutes) coincides with the point at which most patients would normally be expected to be fit for discharge after a single dose of midazolam.

Allergy to the benzodiazepines is rare. However, as the common core structure of these drugs is almost identical, a patient who exhibits an allergic reaction to any benzodiazepine must not be managed with flumazenil, which would only worsen the situation.

Mechanism of action of benzodiazepines

Benzodiazepines act throughout the CNS. Specific benzodiazepine receptors are located on nerve cells within the brain. All benzodiazepine molecules have a common core shape, which enables them to attach to these receptors. The effect of attaching benzodiazepines to cell membrane receptors is to alter an existing physiological filter.

The normal passage of information from the peripheral senses to the brain is filtered by the GABA (gamma aminobutyric acid) system. GABA is an inhibitory neurotransmitter which is released from sensory nerve endings as a result of nerve stimuli passing from neurone to neurone. When released, GABA attaches to receptors on the cell membrane of the postsynaptic neurone. This stabilises the neurone by increasing the threshold for firing. In this way, the number of sensory messages perceived by the brain is reduced. Benzodiazepine receptors are located on cell membranes close to GABA receptors (Fig 3-9). The effect of having a benzodiazepine in place on a receptor is to prolong the effect of GABA. This further reduces the number of stimuli reaching the higher centres and produces pharmacological sedation, anxiolysis, amnesia, muscle relaxation and anticonvulsant effects. Benzodiazepines must cross the blood–brain barrier to reach their target receptors.

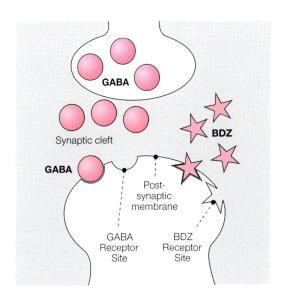

Fig 3-9 GABA (gamma aminobutyric acid) and BDZ (benzodiazepine) receptors.

Highly lipophilic agents such as midazolam reach the CNS receptors quickly and easily.

All benzodiazepines which are CNS depressants have a similar shape with a ring structure on the same position of the diazepine part of each molecule. By contrast, flumazenil, the benzodiazepine antagonist, does not have this ring structure and has a neutral effect on the GABA system. Flumazenil is an effective antagonist, as it has a greater affinity for the benzodiazepine receptor than the active drugs and therefore displaces them.

Paradoxical or unusual effects are exhibited by some patients when sedated with benzodiazepines. Patients who misuse CNS active drugs are often difficult to sedate. This may be due to altered activity at the receptor level. This may be manifest as failure to achieve sedation, an unusually short period of effective sedation or hyperactivity. The greater sensitivity to even small doses of drug seen in older people may be the result of a reduction in the number or effectiveness of CNS receptors and/or a slower circulation. For this reason, the rate of titration and the size of the increments must be reduced.

Metabolism of benzodiazepines occurs in the liver. Some drugs are broken down to metabolites which have a longer elimination half-life than the parent drug. An example of this is diazepam. Diazepam is degraded to several metabolites including desmethyldiazepam, which has sedative properties and a half-life of several days. Midazolam has no metabolites which are active once the parent drug has been eliminated. This is a major advantage of midazolam and is the principal reason for its being considered the drug of choice for outpatient conscious sedation. The water-soluble metabolites of the benzodiazepines are excreted via the kidneys.

The anterograde amnesia produced is a desirable effect in terms of reducing the patient's memory of treatment but, paradoxically, is less helpful when trying to "wean" patients away from treatment under sedation. It is important to remember that there is no loss of memory of events which take place before the injection of midazolam. The most profound amnesia occurs immediately after induction, but some disturbance to short-term memory may persist for several hours or even until the following day. Midazolam-induced amnesia may be prolonged. It is therefore essential to warn both patients and their escorts of this possibility. It is advisable not to guarantee complete amnesia as this effect varies between patients and in the same patient on different occasions. The effect of anterograde amnesia is often misinterpreted by patients with the result that they believe that they have been unconscious. This may lead to difficulties. When the patient returns for treatment under sedation they may insist that they are under-sedated or more awake than before.

The muscle relaxant effect of benzodiazepines contributes to the difficulty in standing, walking or maintaining balance experienced by many patients following treatment.

Respiratory Effects

Benzodiazepines produce respiratory depression. This is usually mild in healthy patients if the drug is administered intravenously by slow titration. It can, however, be a significant problem in unwell or elderly people. Even in a fit healthy individual, a fast injection or a large quantity of midazolam has the potential to depress respiration to the point of apnoea.

There are two mechanisms by which ventilation is depressed. First, relaxation of the muscles of respiration causes a dose-related reduction in the rate and depth of breathing. Second, the reduction in sensitivity of the central carbon dioxide and oxygen chemoreceptors decreases the ability of the respiratory centre to increase the respiratory drive in the presence of hypercarbia and/or hypoxia (see Chapter 2).

Benzodiazepine-induced respiratory depression affects all patients who are sedated with these drugs by any route of administration. For this reason it is important to monitor respiration throughout sedation particularly with intravenous sedation but also after the oral administration of benzodiazepines. Respiration should be monitored clinically by observation of the rate and depth of breathing; however, since it is not always easy to detect small changes in respiratory function a pulse oximeter is mandatory.

Cardiovascular Effects

Benzodiazepines have few significant cardiovascular effects in healthy people. There is a decrease in mean arterial pressure, cardiac output, stroke volume and systemic vascular resistance. This may present as a small fall in arterial blood pressure immediately following induction of sedation. However, this is normally compensated by the baroreceptor reflex and is of negligible clinical significance except in people with compromising cardiovascular disease.

Propofol

Propofol (Diprivan® 1%) is a synthetic phenol anaesthetic induction agent which was introduced for clinical use in the late 1970s (Fig 3-10). It is the induction agent of choice for day-case surgery due to its rapid onset, short duration and fast recovery.

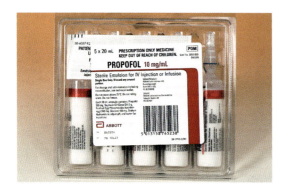

Fig 3-10 Propofol ampoules (200 mg/20 ml).

Propofol: Properties

Injection characteristics	*Painful in small veins*
Anxiolysis	*Yes*
Cardiorespiratory stability	*Stable*
Ease of titration	*Infusion*
Induction and recovery rate	*Very rapid*
Metabolism	*Yes*
Potency	*High*
Speed of change in sedation level	*Very rapid*
Reversibility	*No*
Systemic toxicity	*Low*
Storage/shelf-life	*Stable/long*
Analgesia	*No*

Propofol is extremely lipid soluble but virtually insoluble in water. Like Diazemuls it is solubilised in an oil–in–water emulsion. Each 20 ml ampoule contains 200 mg of propofol (10 mg/ml). The solution is sometimes painful on injection particularly when a small vein is used. However, injecting into a large vein and/or adding 1 ml of 1% plain lidocaine (approximately 0.1 mg/kg) to each 20 ml (200 mg) of propofol helps to reduce pain.

The pharmacokinetics of propofol which make it an ideal agent for day–case general anaesthesia also make it suitable, in lower doses, for sedation. The redistribution half–life is approximately two to four minutes. In order to maintain sedation at a constant level, it is therefore necessary to administer propofol by continuous infusion. Metabolism takes place in the liver and metabolites of propofol are excreted by the kidneys. The elimination half–life is about 60 minutes in fit patients.

Propofol is very useful for short procedures when sedation is required for only a few minutes, for example, for the extraction of a single tooth. Recovery occurs rapidly after the drug is discontinued. The short redistribution half–life prevents the accumulation of drug in the body and, as a consequence, propofol is also an appropriate agent for much longer cases – for example, implant surgery.

There has been some discussion in the literature as to the appropriateness of using propofol in people with epilepsy. Propofol has been reported to be capable of inducing grand mal seizures in patients with no history of epilepsy. Conversely, propofol has also been used to suppress convulsions! Until this situation is clarified, it is wise to avoid selecting this drug for patients with any history of epilepsy.

As with midazolam, propofol tends to depress respiration. The frequency of hypersensitivity reactions is similar to that of other anaesthetic induction agents.

Opioids

For some patients, the use of a single agent does not provide an adequate degree of sedation to enable treatment to be provided. In these cases a combination of agents may make treatment possible, thereby avoiding the need for general anaesthesia. The most frequently used combination of agents is an opioid and midazolam. Individual opioids, like benzodiazepines, act through CNS receptors and have either agonist or antagonistic actions. These drugs produce a number of therapeutic effects including analgesia, sedation

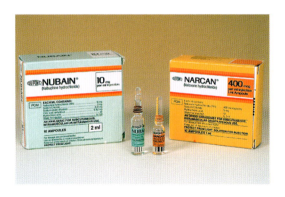

Fig 3-11 Nalbuphine (10 mg/ml) and naloxone (400 micrograms/ml).

and euphoria. Their undesirable effects include cardiorespiratory depression and nausea and vomiting. The most important of these in relation to conscious sedation is respiratory depression. Great care must always be taken when a combination of an opioid and a benzodiazepine is used for sedation. In dental sedation the most frequently used opioid is nalbuphine but fentanyl and its derivatives are also used. Nalbuphine (Nubain®) has the advantage that it is not a controlled drug and so, unlike other opioids, special security precautions are not required.

Nalbuphine (Fig 3-11) must be given before midazolam is titrated. The incidence of vomiting is about 30% with this technique – it is sometimes necessary to administer an antiemetic.

If any opioid is used for sedation the opioid antagonist naloxone (Narcan®) must be available (Fig 3-11). Naloxone is a pure opioid antagonist and reverses respiratory depression, analgesia and sedation.

Inhalational Agents

Inhalational agents are commonly used for dental sedation. Traditionally nitrous oxide has been the only gas used, but volatile anaesthetic agents are now being investigated and may have a role to play in the future. No currently available agent is ideal. The greatest potential danger when using inhalational sedation is the failure to deliver an adequate supply of oxygen to the patient, due to inappropriate or faulty equipment. No correctly maintained Relative Analgesia machine should be capable of administering less than 30% oxygen.

Properties of an Ideal Inhalational Sedation Agent

Induction characteristics	Smooth
Anxiolysis	Yes
Cardiorespiratory stability	Stable
Ease of titration	Easy
Induction and recovery rate	Rapid
Metabolism	0%
Ease of breathing	Non-pungent
Blood gas solubility	Low
Potency (MAC)	Weak (high)
Speed of change in sedation level	Rapid
Systemic toxicity	None
Environmental effects	None
Analgesia	Yes

The minimum alveolar concentration (MAC) is a value obtained experimentally which represents the potency of an inhalational agent. A high MAC indicates an agent of low potency which is ideal for conscious sedation.

Nitrous oxide

Nitrous oxide is rapidly absorbed. The rate of absorption depends on a number of factors, including the solubility of the drug in blood. Agents with low solubility produce rapid onset of sedation because the concentration of drug in blood, and therefore in the brain, rapidly equilibrates with the inspired concentration. When the agent is discontinued, recovery occurs quickly as the concentration of the agent falls. Nitrous oxide has a high MAC compared with most volatile anaesthetic agents.

The nitrous oxide molecule is excreted unchanged almost exclusively by the lungs. It is therefore suitable for patients with (even advanced) liver or kidney disease. It has little effect on the respiratory system as it is non-irritant and does not increase bronchial secretions or depress respiration centrally. The cardiovascular effects of nitrous oxide are insignificant in healthy patients. The inspired concentration of nitrous oxide at which sedation occurs varies

Properties of Nitrous Oxide

Induction characteristics	Smooth
Anxiolysis	Yes
Cardiorespiratory stability	Stable
Ease of titration	Easy
Induction and recovery rate	Rapid
Metabolism	<1%
Ease of breathing	Non-pungent
Potency (MAC)	Weak (105%)
Blood gas solubility	Low (0.47)
Speed of change in sedation level	Rapid
Systemic toxicity	Yes (prolonged use)
Environmental effects	Yes
Analgesia	Yes

from patient to patient. In some people 70% nitrous oxide has no effect whereas in others (especially the elderly) 25% may produce unconsciousness, with loss of airway-protective reflexes. Traditionally, three planes of Relative Analgesia are described (Table 3-2). Planes I and II are clinically useful for dental sedation. Plane III is generally considered to be too close to anaesthesia to be safe in the dental outpatient setting.

The low solubility of nitrous oxide in blood and tissues results in a rapid out-flow of nitrous oxide across the alveolar membrane when the incoming gas flow is stopped (Fig 3-12). This reduces the percentage of alveolar oxygen available for. This phenomenon – "diffusion hypoxia" – may be counter-acted by giving 100% oxygen for two minutes at the end of the procedure.

In the UK, nitrous oxide is supplied in blue cylinders containing both gaseous and liquid phases under high pressure (5400 kPa or 800 psi).

Table 3-2 Planes of relative analgesia.

Planes	Definition
Plane I	moderate sedation and analgesia. usually obtained with concentrations of 5–25% N_2O
Plane II	dissociation sedation and analgesia usually obtained with concentrations of 20–55% N_2O
Plane III	total analgesia usually obtained with concentrations of 50–70% N_2O

N_2O, nitrous oxide.

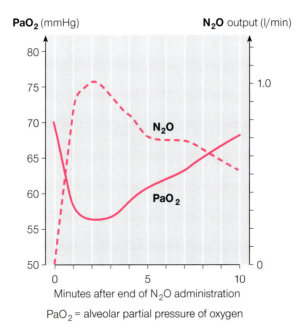

Fig 3-12 Diffusion hypoxia.

Disadvantages of Nitrous Oxide

Long-term occupational (or recreational) exposure to nitrous oxide is an area of increasing concern. Biochemical, haematological, neurological and reproductive side effects have been reported.

Nitrous oxide produces reversible inhibition of the enzyme methionine synthetase which is involved in the synthesis of vitamin B_{12}. Clinically significant bone marrow depression can be detected after six hours' exposure to 60% nitrous oxide (or after much lower percentages for much longer periods of time). Nitrous oxide has also been linked to an increase in the rate of miscarriage among women dentists and dental nurses.

Effective waste gas scavenging appears to reduce the risks and daily exposure to very low concentrations (<100 ppm). Under such circumstances, nitrous oxide is unlikely to cause any serious problems (see Chapter 6). There are also concerns about the possible harmful effects of nitrous oxide on the environment, notably the ozone-depleting greenhouse gas effect.

Sevoflurane
Sevoflurane is a fluorinated derivative of methyl isopropyl ether which was first synthesised in the early 1970s.

Sevoflurane: Properties

Induction characteristics	Smooth
Anxiolysis	Yes
Cardiorespiratory stability	Stable
Ease of titration	Easy
Induction and recovery rate	Rapid
Metabolism	5%
Ease of breathing	Non-pungent
Blood gas solubility	Low (0.6)
Potency (MAC)	High (2%)
Speed of change in sedation level	Fairly rapid
Systemic toxicity	None known
Environmental effects	Minimal
Analgesia	No

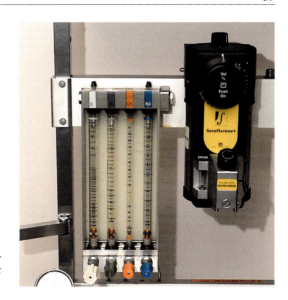

Fig 3-13 Sevoflurane vaporiser mounted on anaesthetic machine.

Sevoflurane is a relatively new anaesthetic agent in the UK, despite it having been used in Japan since the early 1980s. It has a MAC of 2% and low blood gas solubility (0.6). These physical characteristics make sevoflurane a potent anaesthetic agent with rapid uptake and speedy recovery. It is used extensively in day-case surgery where rapid recovery is important. It is pleasant to inhale, non-irritant and non-pungent.

The properties that make sevoflurane a useful anaesthetic agent also make it a promising sedation agent. However, a specially calibrated vaporiser (Fig 3-13) is required in order to titrate low concentrations of sevoflurane (up to 1%) in oxygen (or nitrous oxide and oxygen). Sevoflurane is partly metabolised (5%) and so some care is required in people with severe liver or kidney disease.

At present sevoflurane is not widely used for dental sedation because of the practical problems associated with attaching a vaporiser to any of the currently available inhalational sedation machines. However, this situation may change if research shows that sevoflurane has significant advantages over nitrous oxide or pollution issues result in the withdrawal of nitrous oxide, as has happened in parts of the USA.

Conclusion

• When selecting sedative drugs, it is important to know and understand their clinical effects. This is the key to safe, effective conscious sedation.

Further Reading

Craig DC, Debuse DC. Sedation drugs and safe practice. Independent Dent 1999;4:78–82.

McCaughey W, Clarke RSJ, Fee JPH, Wallace WFM (Eds.). Anaesthetic Physiology and Pharmacology. London: Churchill Livingstone, 1997.

Chapter 4

Initial Assessment and Treatment Planning

Aim

The aim of this chapter is to describe the principles of assessment and treatment planning for patients undergoing conscious sedation.

Outcome

After reading this chapter you should have an understanding of the importance of pre-sedation assessment and the factors that influence treatment planning for patients undergoing conscious sedation.

Introduction

The assessment of the anxious dental patient is probably one of the most important and challenging aspects of everyday clinical practice. Unless a reasonable rapport is achieved at this stage and the patient perceives that the dental team is "on their side", there is a risk that subsequent treatment may fail, no matter how hard one tries, or which conscious sedation technique is used. Many patients expect dental treatment to be uncomfortable and even painful. These concerns may cause reactions which range from mild apprehension, through various degrees of anxiety to irrational fear (phobia). Both pain and anxiety should be adequately controlled to minimise the risk of adverse physiological effects resulting from these psychological responses. The risk of an adverse event is increased in individuals with medical conditions and in elderly patients.

Any social or medical problem represents a departure from normal and may require modifications in treatment planning. This may involve simply a change in attitude on the part of the practitioner or a more significant alteration in the scheduling of dental care. In all events, it is important to match the patient's ability to cope with treatment and the pace of delivery. In particular, vulnerable patients require positive management rather than being denied good quality care. For example, people with learning disabilities will require more information and more time, often involving other professionals and family or carers.

The principal role of conscious sedation is to allay apprehension, anxiety or fear. It is also used to reduce the stress associated with traumatic or prolonged procedures (e.g. implant surgery) and/or to control gagging. Additionally, conscious sedation is beneficial in stabilising the blood pressure in patients with hypertension or a history of cardiovascular or cerebrovascular disease. To be able to recognise individuals who would benefit from conscious sedation, the dental team must be sensitive to the typical signs and symptoms of anxiety.

Signs of anxiety:
- clenched fists
- sweaty hands
- pallor
- distracted appearance
- sitting forward in the dental chair
- holding handbag/tissue tightly
- persistent talking and interruption or silent demeanour
- frequent throat clearing
- constant looking around
- not smiling
- restlessness and fidgeting
- licking lips
- aggressive behaviour.

Symptoms of anxiety:
- dry mouth
- need to visit lavatory
- nausea (and vomiting)
- fainting
- tiredness
- sweating.

The Assessment Visit

A satisfactory first visit is crucial to the success of subsequent treatment under sedation. This meeting should ideally not be in the surgery environment and should be in the nature of an informal "chat". Many patients feel unable to attend on their own. A supportive accompanying relative or friend may make the assessment easier for both the patient and the dentist. However, not all accompanying persons are helpful and some may actually hinder the process. Beware the husband or wife who does not allow their spouse to answer your questions without interruption! It is often easy to spot the relative who will best help the patient by remaining in the waiting room during the assessment interview. Young children are a special case and should never be assessed without a parent or carer present.

There is a great deal of information to be acquired from the patient and so it is important to have a structured approach. Since patients often become more relaxed as the interview proceeds, it is advisable to defer any questions which may be perceived as threatening until the patient is more relaxed. It should never be forgotten that the patient is also assessing the operator during this interview.

The following areas need to be explored during the initial assessment.

What is the Problem?

It is often helpful to get the patient to complete a questionnaire about the nature of their fears. Suitable questionnaires for adults include the Modified Dental Anxiety Scale (Fig 4-1) and for children the Venham Scale (Fig 4-2). These serve to break the ice and allow other lines of questioning to be introduced. It is not helpful to encourage the patient to relive and recall a series of unsatisfactory dental experiences. Remember, for some patients discussing dentistry can be frightening! Rather, the dentist should steer the conversation towards positive solutions whilst reassuring the individual that their concerns are being taken seriously. It is unwise, however, to be drawn into promising too much too soon, in relation to the benefits of sedation, or the extent of dental treatment that may be provided. Many anxious patients have unrealistic expectations. Unless this is resolved at an early stage, it is likely that patients will be dissatisfied if treatment does not progress as they would have liked.

Medical History and Investigations

It is essential that a comprehensive medical history is obtained by the dentist. This takes time to record properly and should not be rushed or delegated to another member of the dental team. If a patient has completed a medical history form before coming to the practice, this must be thoroughly checked and any significant areas investigated. It is not acceptable to rely solely on the information provided by an apprehensive patient, as their state of mind may result in the withholding of important details.

The Modified Dental Anxiety Scale

Can you tell us how anxious you get, if at all, with your dental visit?
Please indicate by inserting "X" in the appropriate box

1. If you went to your dentist for **TREATMENT TOMORROW**, how would you feel?

Not anxious ☐   Slightly anxious ☐   Fairly anxious ☐   Very anxious ☐   Extremely anxious ☐

2. If you were sitting in the **WAITING ROOM** (waiting for treatment), how would you feel?

Not anxious ☐   Slightly anxious ☐   Fairly anxious ☐   Very anxious ☐   Extremely anxious ☐

3. If you were about to have a **TOOTH DRILLED**, how would you feel?

Not anxious ☐   Slightly anxious ☐   Fairly anxious ☐   Very anxious ☐   Extremely anxious ☐

4. If you were about to have you **TEETH SCALED AND POLISHED**, how would you feel?

Not anxious ☐   Slightly anxious ☐   Fairly anxious ☐   Very anxious ☐   Extremely anxious ☐

5. If you were about to have a **LOCAL ANAESTHETIC INJECTION** in your gum, how would you feel?

Not anxious ☐   Slightly anxious ☐   Fairly anxious ☐   Very anxious ☐   Extremely anxious ☐

Fig 4-1 Modified Dental Anxiety Scale.

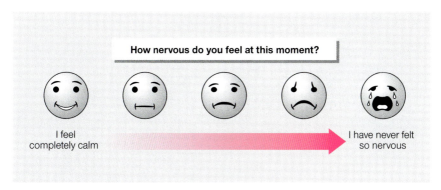

Fig 4-2 Venham Scale of Anxiety.

From the sedation point of view, special note should be made of respiratory and cardiovascular problems and liver and kidney diseases. Prescribed medication may alert the operator to undisclosed medical conditions and also raise the question of possible drug interactions.

Pregnancy (confirmed or possible) is generally considered to be a contraindication to the elective use of sedation with benzodiazepines. Nitrous oxide is best avoided in the first trimester. Mothers who are breast feeding must be advised that benzodiazepines may be passed to their baby through their milk.

Some medicines potentiate the effect of sedation drugs and vice versa. Where there is doubt, it is sensible to discuss the patient's medical history with their general medical practitioner or consultant. This must be done with the consent of the patient. It should be noted that there are very few drugs which absolutely contraindicate the concurrent use of benzodiazepines or nitrous oxide. Patients taking (or using) drugs which depress the CNS often sedate unpredictably. Provided that the sedative agent is titrated to a satisfactory sedation end-point there are usually no significant adverse effects. Although allergy to benzodiazepines is very rare, if there is any suggestion of a previous reaction to any drugs in this group, the patient should undergo allergy testing or an alternative agent should be used.

A full medical examination is not usually necessary, but the sedationist should make an overall assessment of the clothed patient for signs of ill health. The following should be noted:

- extremes of weight
- gait, use of walking stick
- airway abnormalities
- breathing difficulties
- cyanosis
- jaundice
- pallor
- prostheses including hearing aids.

Baseline recordings of heart rate and arterial blood pressure should be obtained and the results recorded in the patient's notes (Figs 4-3–4-5).

Having collected this information it is now possible to assess the operative and/or sedation risk according to the scale of physical fitness devised by the American Society of Anesthesiologists (ASA) (Table 4-1).

Patients classified as ASA I or II are generally considered suitable for treatment in general dental practice or other primary dental care settings. Those falling into categories III and IV should be referred to a specialist centre such as a teaching hospital or specialist sedation clinic. Some patients oscillate back and forth between ASA III and ASA IV according to the severity of their disease and other factors such as the season of the year. Examples of this type of fluctuating conditions include: poorly controlled asthma, diabetes mellitus and epilepsy. It may be preferable to refer such patients for specialist care or wait until their condition becomes more stable before providing treatment under sedation.

Table 4-1 ASA fitness scale.

Scale	Description
I	normal healthy patients
II	patients with mild systemic disease
III	patients with severe systemic disease that is limiting but not incapacitating
IV	patients with incapacitating disease that is a constant threat to life
V	patients not expected to live more than 24 hours

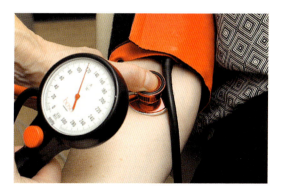

Fig 4-3 Aneroid sphygmo-manometer and stethoscope.

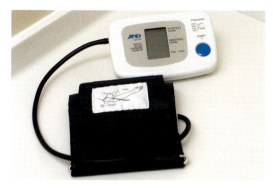

Fig 4-4 Electronic sphyg-momanometer.

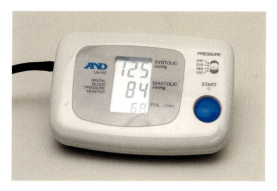

Fig 4-5 Electronic sphyg-momanometer display.

Dental History

The patient's experiences at the dentist over the years are important. The following questions may yield valuable information which will be helpful during treatment planning:

- Are there any current symptoms (particularly pain)?
- Has "normal" dentistry been possible in the past?
- When did dental anxiety start?
- What provoked the fear?
- When did the patient last visit a dentist?
- Has the patient had treatment under sedation in the past?
- If so, what kind of sedation?
- Was this treatment successful?
- What concerns the patient most about their teeth?
- What treatment does the patient want?

If the patient has been referred by another practitioner (either medical or dental) it is important to distinguish between what the referring practitioner has requested and what the patient really wants. For example, a patient referred for extensive periodontal treatment of a large number of uncomfortable, unattractive and very mobile teeth may actually prefer a treatment plan involving extractions and the provision of dentures!

Social Factors

It is always important to enquire about a patient's domestic circumstances:
- Is an escort available?
- Is the escort a responsible adult?
- If required, can the escort remain with the patient overnight?
- If not, what alternative arrangements are there?
- Can the patient take sufficient time off work?
- Does the patient have other responsibilities (childcare, care of elderly, etc.)
- How difficult is the journey to and from the practice?

Social factors assume a larger degree of importance when conscious sedation techniques are used compared with the provision of routine dental care. Perversely, many patients who present with difficult dental problems also have social problems – for example, homelessness, alcohol and drug dependence. These can complicate management and aftercare.

Dental Examination

Whilst some anxious patients will tolerate a full intraoral examination, the operator may have to be content with only a visual examination at this stage. Many patients particularly dislike the dental probe and so this instrument should only be used when absolutely necessary, and then with extreme caution. For a few patients, intraoral radiographs may also be threatening or cause gagging and may have to be carried out when the patient returns for treatment under sedation.

At this stage, one should aim to gain an overview of the patient's treatment needs and to identify a suitable starting point. It is wise not to plan extensive treatment for the first visit except when the patient is in pain. A small restoration, simple extraction or scaling may be most appropriate.

Treatment Planning

During the initial visit, only a preliminary treatment plan can be formulated, as it is impossible to predict how any individual patient will be able to cooperate with treatment under conscious sedation. An extensive or complex treatment plan promised in advance may falsely raise both the dentist's and the patient's expectations.

The following options for the management of pain and anxiety may then be considered and discussed with the patient:
• local anaesthesia alone
• local anaesthesia with inhalational sedation
• local anaesthesia with intravenous sedation
• local anaesthesia with oral sedation.

The simplest technique which will enable treatment to be carried out is generally considered to be the most appropriate. It is not appropriate to subject patients to a rigid cascade of management options by only being prepared to consider more complex forms of sedation when all simpler techniques have failed. This is unnecessarily distressing for patients (and the dental team) and may serve to increase anxiety and reduce willingness to cooperate. For example, a severely anxious patient with needle phobia who requires extensive dentistry may benefit most from the prescription of high-dose oral benzodiazepine sedation from the outset. Coercing such a patient to submit to venepuncture or inhalational sedation, knowing that these are very likely to fail, is bad practice.

Written consent is required for both the dental procedure and the administration of conscious sedation. Consent for dentistry under conscious sedation should, wherever possible, be broad enough to allow both examination and the provision of routine treatment. If extractions or advanced procedures are required, these must be agreed on a tooth-by-tooth basis. This is not practical for routine restorative dentistry. Finally, patients must be given written and verbal pre- and postoperative instructions and have the opportunity to ask questions.

Patient Instructions for Conscious Sedation

For your safety, please read and follow these instructions carefully

BEFORE SEDATION: ON THE DAY OF TREATMENT

Take your routine medicines at the usual times

Have only light meals and non-alcoholic drinks on the day of your appointment

Bring a responsible adult with you – someone who is able to escort you home and then care for you for the rest of the day

AFTER SEDATION: UNTIL THE FOLLOWING DAY

Do not travel alone – travel home with your escort, by car if possible

Do not drive or ride a bicycle

Do not operate machinery

Do not drink alcohol

Do not return to work or sign legal documents

The First Sedation Visit

The purpose of the first sedation appointment is to:
- assess the efficacy of conscious sedation
- complete a thorough oral and dental examination
- relieve pain
- formulate a potentially achievable dental treatment plan.

At the end of this appointment the broad aims of the proposed dental treatment should be discussed with the patient in the presence of their escort so that both are aware of what will take place at the next visit. Since the patient will still be under the influence of the sedative agent at this time, a more detailed discussion will be needed before the administration of sedation at the second visit. If this first appointment has not gone as well as was hoped, an honest explanation should be given to the patient and their escort and consideration given to changing the sedation technique and/or adjusting the treatment aims. For example, a patient who is only just manageable under intravenous sedation may be better served by extractions and the provision of a partial denture rather than a heroic attempt to restore broken-down teeth.

Conclusions

- Assessment is important before providing conscious sedation.
- Treatment planning is tailored by the patient's response to sedation.

Further Reading

Corah N, Gale E, Illig S. Assessment of a dental anxiety scale. J Dent Res 1978;97:816–819.

Debuse DC, Craig DC. Conscious sedation in dentistry. Independent Dent 1998;3:60–62.

Humphris G, Morrison T, Lindsay S. The Modified Dental Anxiety Scale: validation and United Kingdom norms. Community Dent Health 1995;12:143–150.

Venham L. The effect of mother's presence on child's response to dental treatment. J Dent Child 1979;46:219–225.

Chapter 5
Equipment for Conscious Sedation

Aim

The aim of this chapter is to describe the equipment required for the administration of conscious sedation and other essential items such as patient monitoring devices.

Outcome

After reading this chapter you should be familiar with the equipment used during conscious sedation in primary dental care.

Inhalational Sedation

All modern inhalational Relative Analgesia (RA) machines are derived from simple anaesthetic machines. They are modified to ensure a minimum concentration of 30% oxygen at all times, which makes them safe for use by a sedationist who is concurrently carrying out the dental treatment. A variety of different commercial models are available. All have similar operational principles and safety features (Figs 5-1 and 5-2).

Gas supply

The gas supply to Relative Analgesia machines may be provided by cylinders mounted below the Relative Analgesia head on a mobile support. In surgeries where several Relative Analgesia units are installed, a pipeline system which supplies gas from a remote tank or large cylinder storage area may be more practical.

Nitrous oxide (N_2O) is supplied in a blue cylinder containing both a gas and liquid phase at a pressure of 5400 kPa (800 psi). Oxygen (O_2) comes as compressed gas in a black cylinder with a white shoulder at a pressure of 15,000 kPa (2000 psi).

Most free-standing inhalational sedation machines are designed to operate with two nitrous oxide and two oxygen cylinders. One cylinder of each gas is designated "IN USE" whilst the other is held in reserve and designated

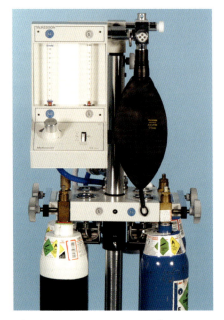 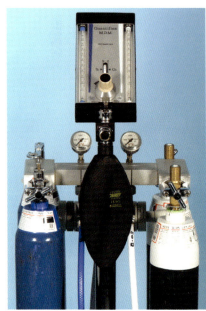

Fig 5-1 McKesson RA machine.   **Fig 5-2** Matrx MDM RA machine.

"FULL". During administration of Relative Analgesia only the "IN USE" cylinder for each gas should be turned on.

The Pin Index System is a safety feature designed to ensure that gas cylinders are correctly mounted on mobile Relative Analgesia machines. This system prevents the accidental interchange of nitrous oxide and oxygen cylinders. Each gas cylinder has two holes drilled into the valve block which exactly match pins on the machine's manifold or yoke (Fig 5-3). The pattern of holes and corresponding pins is unique for each gas (Figs 5-4 and 5-5).

The gas-tight fit between each cylinder and the machine is dependent upon the presence of an intact seal between the face of the valve block and the manifold. This is provided by a small (but vital) piece of equipment, the Bodok seal (Fig 5-6). Absence of any one of the four Bodok seals renders the whole machine unserviceable.

The nitrous oxide and oxygen pressure gauges give an indication of the liquid and gas remaining in each cylinder. Whilst the oxygen gauge falls continuously in a linear manner as the gas is used, the nitrous oxide gauge will

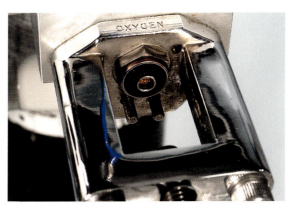

Fig 5-3 Yoke for attachment of gas cylinder.

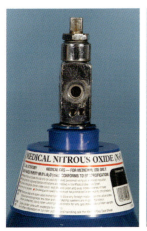

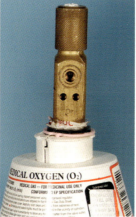

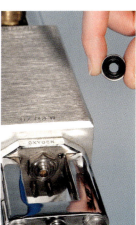

Fig 5-4 Pin Index pattern for nitrous oxide. **Fig 5-5** Pin Index pattern for oxygen. **Fig 5-6** Bodok seal.

only begin to fall from its maximum reading when all the liquid has been converted to gas. This is because the nitrous oxide cylinder contains both liquid and gas phases and full pressure is maintained until this point.

Pressure-reducing valves located underneath the top plate of the machine reduce the relatively high cylinder pressures to 413 kPa (60 psi) (Fig 5-7). The gases then pass to the head of the machine via colour-coded, non–interchangeable NIST (National Institute of Science and Technology) pipelines.

61

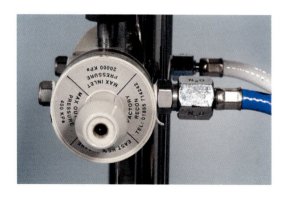

Fig 5-7 Pressure-reducing valve.

Relative Analgesia machine "heads" comprise flow meters for nitrous oxide and oxygen, a control valve for regulating the total gas flow and a mixture dial for adjusting the percentage of oxygen and nitrous oxide (Figs 5-8–5-10). All modern machines are incapable of delivering a gas mixture containing less than 30% oxygen. They are also equipped with a failsafe mechanism which shuts off the nitrous oxide if oxygen ceases to flow. The head has an oxygen flush button and an air entrainment valve which opens if the mixed gas supply fails.

Mixed oxygen and nitrous oxide emerges at the common gas outlet to which the patient breathing system is connected. A 2 litre reservoir bag is also attached at the common gas outlet (Fig 5-11). This is used for adjusting the total gas flow to each individual patient's minute volume requirement and for monitoring respiration during treatment. Reservoir bags are made of antistatic rubber and are liable to perish, especially in the area of the bag mount (neck).

Although there are many designs, all modern Relative Analgesia breathing systems comprise an inspiratory limb (tube), a nasal mask and an expiratory limb. Systems for use with active scavenging differ from those for use with passive removal of waste gases (Figs 5-12 and 5-13). Active scavenging is achieved by connecting the expiratory limb of the breathing system to a low power suction device whilst passive scavenging often involves nothing more than hanging the end of the tube out of a convenient window.

Relative Analgesia masks are supplied in a variety of sizes (Fig 5-14) and different designs (Figs 5-15 and 5-16) depending upon whether they are to be

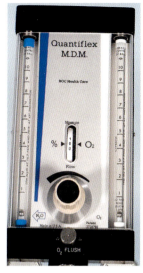

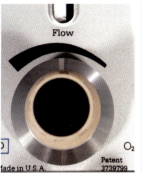

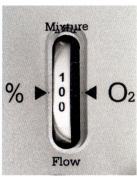

Fig 5-9 Gas flow control. **Fig 5-10** Gas mixture dial.

Fig 5-8 Matrx MDM machine head.

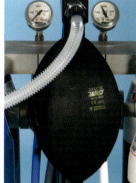

Fig 5-11 Reservoir bag (2 litres).

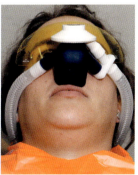

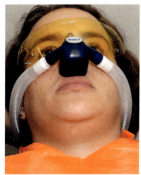

Fig 5-12 Active scavenging mask assembly. **Fig 5-13** Passive scavenging mask assembly.

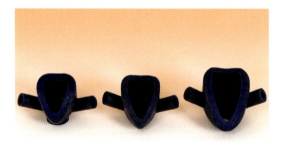

Fig 5-14 Small, medium and large masks.

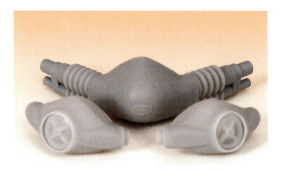

Fig 5-15 Porter scavenging masks.

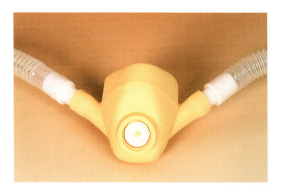

Fig 5-16 Accutron Personal Inhaler.

used with an active or passive scavenging system (Figs 5-17 and 5-18) and whether they are single use or reusable. One system for active scavenging comprises a neoprene mask and plastic mushroom-shaped scavenging disc which is designed to scavenge some of the gas which escapes from the open

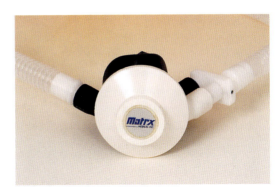

Fig 5-17 Matrx active scavenging mask.

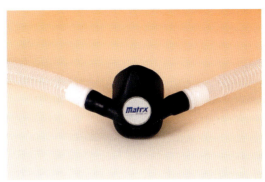

Fig 5-18 Matrx passive scavenging mask.

mouth during treatment. These two parts have to be fitted together before use. Note that the expiratory limb of the breathing system is fitted into the rubber connector on the "mushroom" whilst the blanked-off tube of the Y piece is attached to the mask section. Older masks and breathing systems may only be cold sterilised. Recent improvements in materials make some newer models suitable for autoclaving. Others are for single use only. Check with your supplier if in doubt.

The older type of breathing system which has an expiratory valve mounted on the nasal mask should never be used. With this system, nitrous oxide is expired directly into the breathing zone of the chairside team.

Environmental nitrous oxide monitors are readily available. These vary from simple lapel sensors (similar to radiation monitors) to complex and expensive devices designed for research purposes.

Equipment checking

A number of checks must be completed before using the Relative Analgesia machine. No compromise on the condition or function of a component can be accepted.

> ### Relative Analgesia machine checklist
>
> ❏ *Cylinders: "FULL" and "IN USE"*
>
> ❏ *Pressure gauges*
>
> ❏ *All connections*
>
> ❏ *Flow and mixture controls*
>
> ❏ *Oxygen flush control*
>
> ❏ *Reservoir bag*
>
> ❏ *Breathing system and range of masks*
>
> ❏ *Scavenging system*

Intravenous Sedation Using Midazolam

The equipment needed for the administration of intravenous midazolam is simple and inexpensive (Fig 5-19). The following are required:
- midazolam
- flumazenil
- syringes (5 ml)
- drawing-up needles (21 gauge)
- cannulae (25 – 21 gauge)
- gauze
- tourniquet
- antiseptic wipes
- stopwatch/clock
- non–allergenic tape
- cotton wool rolls
- plasters.

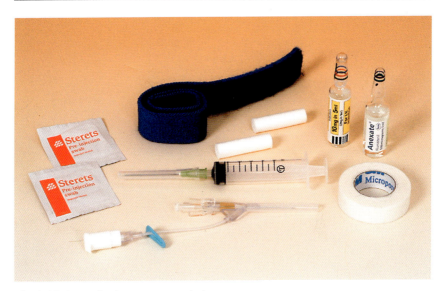

Fig 5-19 Items for intravenous sedation.

Drugs and syringes

The most useful size of syringe is 5 ml. This is ideal for midazolam presented as 10 mg in 5 ml (and also for flumazenil which is presented as 500 microgams in 5 ml). However, some practitioners favour the 10 mg in 2 ml concentration of midazolam which is best administered with a 2 ml syringe. Note that the latter, a more concentrated solution, is much more difficult to titrate due to the very small volume of each increment. Using this preparation, 1 ml of injected solution delivers 5 mg of midazolam, or, put another way, each 1 mg increment requires the accurate injection of only 0.2 ml of the solution.

Some practitioners dilute the standard midazolam solution with sterile water to produce a concentration of 10 mg in 10 ml. This may have the marginal advantage of making drug administration easier for people with limited computational skills who are confused by the idea that each millilitre of solution does NOT contain 1 milligram of midazolam. This practice is not, however, recommended. Changing the manufacturer's concentration of any drug inevitably increases the risk of errors and thus possible adverse effects and accidents.

It is important to ensure that the design of the syringe hub is compatible with both the drawing-up needle (21 gauge is ideal) and the cannula system in

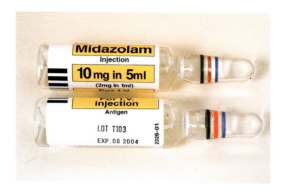

Fig 5-20 Midazolam label detail.

use. In particular, syringes with a Luer-Lok hub cannot be easily and securely attached to some makes of intravenous cannulae.

Before drawing up the sedation drug, the following details must be checked and recorded in the clinical notes (Fig 5-20):
• drug name
• condition of drug and ampoule
• concentration
• volume of solution
• expiry date
• batch number.

A piece of clean gauze is useful to hold the drug ampoule whilst it is opened. This limits the risk of damage to the operator's fingers. Wearing gloves further protects against injury.

Having checked that the correct drug has been drawn up, the syringe must be labelled appropriately. The label should be placed on the syringe barrel so that the operator can still see the graduation markings during injection.

It is considered best practice that all patients undergoing intravenous sedation should have a flexible plastic cannula placed in a vein so as to ensure reliable continuous venous access throughout the procedure (Fig 5-21). Butterfly needles are not recommended as they are more likely to cut through the vein if the patient moves their hand or arm. A further disadvantage is that they usually become occluded by a blood clot some 5–10 minutes after administration of the sedative drug. Cannulae do not present these disadvantages and, contrary to popular belief, are not more difficult or more painful

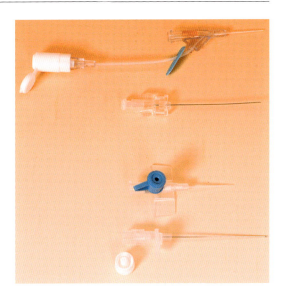

Fig 5-21 Disassembled Y-
Can and Venflon cannulae.

to insert. In a very small number of patients, however, the insertion of a cannula proves, on occasion, to be impossible. In such cases, it is reasonable to
place a butterfly needle to allow the patient to receive the care they need.
The possibility of a blood clot forming within the lumen of the needle can
be reduced by intermittent flushing with sterile saline.

The most suitable sizes of cannulae for conscious sedation are 20, 21 and 23
gauge. The Wallace Y-Can system has the advantage of preventing blood
loss from the proximal end of the cannula as the metal stylet is removed following venepuncture. A tourniquet is applied in order to restrict the venous
return from (but not the arterial supply to) the limb. This engorges the veins
whilst cannulation is performed. Alternatively, an experienced nurse may
be able to perform this in a more sympathetic way. An antiseptic wipe may
be used to cleanse the skin surface prior to venepuncture. This procedure
also increases the visibility of the patient's veins due to dampening of the
skin. Non-allergenic adhesive tape is used both to secure the cannula and,
at the end of the procedure, to hold a dressing (e.g. a dental cotton wool roll)
over the venepuncture site.

A timing device which has a second hand should be available to monitor the
rate of drug titration. Relying on one's own estimate of the passage of time
is notoriously unreliable.

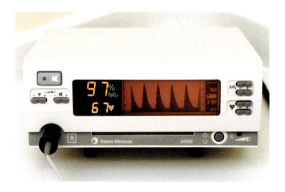

Fig 5-22 Pulse oximeter display.

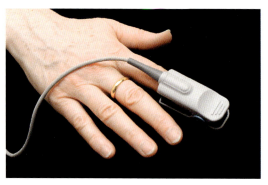

Fig 5-23 Pulse oximeter finger probe.

Pulse Oximetry

Pulse oximeters measure arterial oxygen saturation (SaO_2) and heart rate (Figs 5-22 and 5-23). The use of a pulse oximeter is mandatory for intravenous sedation. It is also essential for oral sedation provided in the dental chair, using temazepam or midazolam. Pulse oximetry is not required during the administration of Relative Analgesia for ASA I/II patients.

Pulse oximeters work by shining a light of known wavelength and intensity through a tissue such as the nail bed of a finger. The amount of light which is absorbed is dependent upon the quantities of reduced haemoglobin and oxyhaemoglobin present in the arterial vascular bed. The pulse oximeter's microprocessor rejects non-pulsatile venous data. The differing light absorption characteristics of oxygenated and non-oxygenated arterial blood are used to compute the SaO_2 continuously.

It is important to remember that the partial pressure of oxygen available to the body tissues is different from and not even directly related to the SaO_2 displayed on the pulse oximeter given the sigmoid shape of the oxygen-haemoglobin dissociation curve (see Chapter 2).

In addition to measuring SaO_2, pulse oximeters display the heart rate. Most pulse oximeters have alarms for low SaO_2, tachycardia and bradycardia. Some models display the arterial plethysmographic (pulse wave) trace, others combine a pulse oximeter with an automatic sphygmomanometer and/or an electrocardiogram.

For dental sedation the SaO_2 alarm limit should be set no lower than 90%. High and low heart rate alarms are normally set at 140 beats per minute and 50 beats per minute respectively.

Pulse oximetry is a simple, non-invasive method of monitoring both the respiratory and the cardiovascular systems and, as such, is probably the single most useful form of monitoring currently available. Absolute reliance should never be placed on any electrical monitoring device. Meticulous clinical monitoring of the patient's condition by both the dentist and the dental nurse remains the most important safeguard of patient safety under sedation.

Equipment for Airway Management

An understanding of the place and use of airway management equipment is also needed by the sedationist. This should not be taken to imply that airway problems are commonplace during conscious sedation for dentistry. There is, of course, a requirement for basic resuscitation equipment to be available in all dental care settings, irrespective of whether or not sedation is practised.

Currently, practitioners using midazolam for intravenous sedation or nitrous oxide and oxygen for inhalational sedation are not required to have been trained in, and have equipment for, the provision of Advanced Life Support (ALS). Nevertheless, many dentists do choose to attend either Advanced or Immediate Life Support (ILS) courses.

The skills and equipment needed for Basic Life Support (BLS), ILS and ALS are defined and regularly reviewed by the Resuscitation Council (UK). The Council's website address is www.resus.org.uk.

Conclusions

- The equipment needed to administer intravenous sedation is simple.
- Important checks must be made on equipment for inhalational sedation before use.
- Monitoring of the sedated patient is essential.

Further Reading

Craig DC, Debuse DC. Equipment for sedation and monitoring. Independent Dent 1998;3:46–52.

Moyle JTB. Principles and Practice Series – Pulse Oximetry. London: BMJ Publishing Group, 1994.

Chapter 6
Clinical Techniques

Aim

This chapter describes the techniques commonly used to sedate patients for treatment in primary care settings.

Outcome

After reading this chapter you should have an understanding of the clinical procedures used during conscious sedation in primary care settings.

Introduction

Inhalation sedation using nitrous oxide and oxygen and intravenous midazolam are by far the most commonly used and useful techniques. Since some appropriately trained and experienced practitioners may use other drugs and routes of administration for selected dental patients, an outline of some alternative techniques is also provided.

There are advantages of having a variety of techniques at one's disposal.
- It allows optimal management of each patient, taking into account medical, psychological and social status. Examples might include a recent history of myocardial infarction, potential interactions with antidepressant medication or domestic or business responsibilities.
- Consideration of the type of dentistry and the length of the intended procedure.
- A combination of techniques may sometimes be appropriate – for example, in a needle-phobic patient for whom nitrous oxide sedation is used to facilitate cannulation for intravenous sedation.

Presedation Preparation

Meticulous preparation will increase the likelihood of success. It is particularly important that the patient is fully prepared for both the sedation and the planned dental procedure. Anxiety is likely to increase if an anxious patient has to wait whilst missing items are found or faulty equipment

Conscious Sedation Techniques

1. In regular use in primary dental care in the UK

   Inhalation sedation (nitrous oxide and oxygen) – Relative analgesia

   Intravenous midazolam

2. Advanced techniques which may only be used by appropriately trained and experienced practitioners

   Intravenous propofol (by infusion)

   Intravenous midazolam plus an opioid

   Oral or intranasal benzodiazepines

replaced. All necessary equipment and drugs must be prepared and checked in advance. When the patient enters the surgery, the dental team must be able to concentrate fully on putting the patient at ease. After the induction of adequate sedation, the dentist must be ready to proceed with treatment without delay. A checklist (Fig 6-1) is a useful aid for training members of the dental team.

The practice environment is also important in putting patients at ease. A quiet, calm environment with minimum interruption provides the best setting for conscious sedation. It is important to avoid having alarming or explicit cardiopulmonary resuscitation posters in full view of anxious patients. This also includes graphic illustrations of florid dental disease or procedures which may increase the level of anxiety in dental phobics. Threatening equipment should also be kept out of site or covered.

Before starting any clinical procedure, it is essential to check the patient's name, medical history and blood pressure. Written consent should have been obtained in advance of the treatment appointment for both the procedure and the sedation. It is also necessary to confirm that the patient has a responsible adult escort who is able and willing to look after the patient for the rest of the day. A patient who does not have a suitable escort should not be sedated. Be wary of patients who say they will "phone a friend" or have

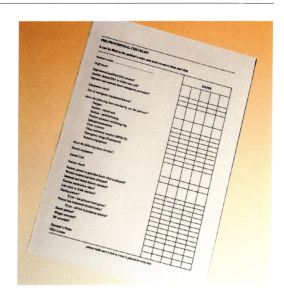

Fig 6-1 Presedation checklist.

arranged a taxi to travel home and then have a neighbour keep an eye on them. These arrangements are never satisfactory, may place the patient at risk and leave the dentist open to criticism if anything goes wrong. If there is any doubt about the quality of aftercare, conscious sedation should NOT be used. A final check should be made to ensure that the appropriate preoperative instructions have been followed and that the patient has been to the lavatory.

Inhalational Sedation with Nitrous Oxide and Oxygen

Nitrous oxide has excellent anxiolytic, sedative and analgesic properties with little or no depression of myocardial function or ventilation. Induction and recovery are rapid. As described in Chapter 3, nitrous oxide has a wide margin of safety.

The response to nitrous oxide sedation varies considerably and unpredictably between patients. One person may be adequately sedated with 20% nitrous oxide, others may require in excess of 50%. A titration technique is therefore employed to avoid the risk of under- or oversedation.

Modern inhalational sedation machines are similar to traditional Boyle's anaesthetic machines, but modified so as to make them safe for use by a seda-

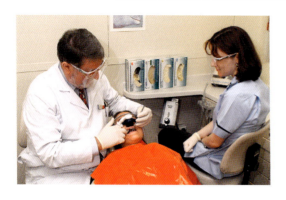

Fig 6-2 Operator-sedationist working with Relative Analgesia.

tionist (see Chapter 5). The inhalational sedation machine must be carefully checked before use. The safety features and ease of operation of purpose-designed inhalation sedation machines make them ideal for a clinician acting as both operator and sedationist (Fig 6-2). Demand-flow devices and equipment designed for general anaesthesia are not suitable for the administration of inhalation sedation by an operator-sedationist. The advantages of inhalational sedation include:

• no needles
• level of sedation easily altered
• minimal impairment of reflexes
• rapid induction and recovery
• some analgesia
• suitable for patients of all ages.

The disadvantages are:

• sedation depends on good psychological support
• postoperative amnesia is variable
• nitrous oxide pollution.

Contraindications of inhalational sedation are:

• nasal obstruction, e.g. cold, polyps, deviated septum
• cyanosis at rest
• poor cooperation
• first trimester (12 weeks) of pregnancy
• fear of masks.

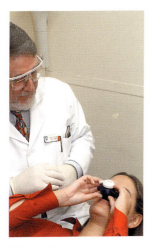
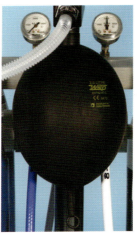
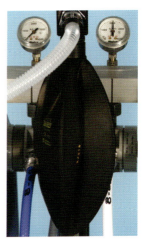

Fig 6-3 Patient trying mask.

Fig 6-4 Overinflated reservoir bag.

Fig 6-5 Underinflated reservoir bag.

Administration of nitrous oxide

After checking that the Relative Analgesia machine is working and that extra gas cylinders are available (or that piped gases are flowing), the patient is laid supine in the chair and the procedure explained. The machine is then adjusted to administer 100% oxygen at a flow rate of 6 litres/min and the correct size nasal mask selected. Patients often prefer to place the mask over their own nose rather than have someone else do it (Fig 6-3). It is important to maintain a steady flow of conversation and encouragement during the induction of sedation. The oxygen flow rate (minute volume) may be checked by observing the movement of the reservoir bag. If there is under- or overinflation of the bag, the gas flow must be increased or decreased respectively (Figs 6-4 and 6-5).

Regular observation of the reservoir bag combined with clinical vital signs provides all the necessary monitoring for fit patients. Pulse oximetry is NOT indicated for ASA I and II patients (see Chapter 4) undergoing inhalation sedation. Patients are receiving a high inspired oxygen concentration continuously and, therefore, arterial oxygen estimations are artificially high. Some practitioners, however, find the continuous heart rate monitoring provided by a pulse oximeter a useful indicator of anxiety.

Ten per cent nitrous oxide is then added (90% oxygen) and the patient informed that he/she may feel:
• lightheaded
• changes in visual/auditory sensation
• tingling of hands and feet
• suffusing warmth
• remote from the immediate environment.

This concentration is maintained for one minute during which verbal encouragement and reassurance are given continuously. The concentration of nitrous oxide is then increased by 10% for a further minute to a total of 20% nitrous oxide. After this, if more sedation is required, increments of 5% nitrous oxide are added per minute until the patient appears and feels sufficiently relaxed.

Nitrous oxide concentrations of between 20% and 50% normally produce a state of detached sedation and analgesia without any loss of consciousness or potential impairment of laryngeal reflexes. At these levels patients are aware of operative procedures and cooperate without being fearful. If, after a period of effective sedation, the patient becomes restless or apprehensive, it is usually the result of disinhibition due to the concentration of nitrous oxide being too high.

Local anaesthesia (LA) should be administered once the patient is sedated. Topical local anaesthesia preparations can be placed during the induction period. The most common cause of apparent failure of nitrous oxide sedation is the assumption that the analgesic properties of nitrous oxide render the use of local anaesthesia unnecessary. This is not the case – nitrous oxide does not provide sufficient analgesia for the majority of dental procedures in either adults or children.

Nitrous oxide has limited solubility in blood and body tissues (see Chapter 3). When the incoming flow of nitrous oxide is stopped there is a rapid outflow of the gas across the alveolar membrane. This may dilute the percentage of alveolar oxygen available for uptake by up to 50%. This phenomenon is called diffusion hypoxia and is prevented by giving 100% oxygen for at least two minutes at the end of the procedure. The patient may then be brought slowly up to the sitting position. Recovery is variable but most patients should be able to walk (with supervision) to a recovery area within five minutes.

All patients, when sufficiently recovered, should be discharged into the care of an escort who must be given written and verbal post-sedation instructions (see Chapter 4). Patients should not be discharged until sufficiently recovered so as to be able to stand and walk without assistance. Recovery is variable and each patient should be individually assessed on every occasion for fitness for discharge. The discharge of patients who have been sedated is the responsibility of the operating dentist.

Nitrous oxide pollution and scavenging

Long-term exposure to nitrous oxide may result in an increased incidence of liver, renal and neurological disease. There is also some evidence of bone marrow toxicity and interference with Vitamin B_{12} synthesis which may lead to signs and symptoms similar to those of pernicious anaemia. In the UK, the Health and Safety Executive specifies a maximum level of 100 ppm of nitrous oxide, time-weighted over eight hours. Scavenging must be employed to safeguard both patients and staff.

Other inhalation sedation methods

In recent years various combinations of isoflurane, desflurane, sevoflurane and oxygen have been investigated. The lack of a suitable delivery system for use by a dental operator-sedationist has slowed development in this area. Sevoflurane shows most promise.

Intravenous Sedation with Midazolam

Midazolam is well suited to conscious sedation for dentistry (Figs 6-6 and 6-7). It is presented in a 5 ml ampoule in a concentration of 2 mg/ml and in a 2 ml ampoule in a concentration of 5 mg/ml. The more dilute presentation (2 mg/ml) is preferred as it is easier to titrate – that is, administer in small increments, whilst observing the patient's response. A titration technique must always be used to reduce the risk of overdosage. It is impossible to determine the correct dosage of midazolam by any form of calculation based on the patient's physical characteristics – for example, age or body weight. Midazolam produces a period of sedation (acute detachment from the individual's surroundings) for 20–30 minutes followed by a state of relaxation for a further hour or so.

Midazolam and anxiolysis: Anxiolysis (dissolving anxiety) is different from sedation and may be described as "dissociating the patient from the perceived threat". It is important to consider the degree of anxiolysis and not just the depth of sedation when assessing the quality of "sedation". An

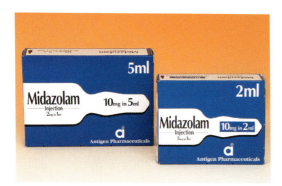

Fig 6-6 Generic midazolam (Antigen).

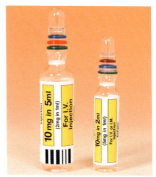

Fig 6-7 Midazolam ampoules (10 mg/5 ml and 10 mg/2 ml).

ideal sedation drug would be anxiolytic rather than sedative, as this would leave the patient fully aware but unconcerned about what was about to happen. Unfortunately, no such drug exists.

With midazolam most patients have little or no recall of the operative procedure. Some patients think they have been anaesthetised rather than sedated, others have difficulty believing that the procedure has already been carried out. This situation must, of course, be fully explained to both the patient and their escort before discharge.

Respiratory depression is seen in all patients undergoing midazolam sedation and is often minimal. There are exceptions – for example, patients with impaired respiratory function or those who have been prescribed (or use) CNS depressant drugs, in particular opioids. Patients may not, of course, admit to recreational drug use. Overdosage and excessively rapid bolus injections often cause profound respiratory depression or possibly even respiratory arrest. The unpredictability of respiratory depression means that a pulse oximeter must always be used whenever intravenous sedation is employed.

The advantages of intravenous midazolam sedation include:
• rapid onset (3–4 minutes or less)
• adequate patient cooperation
• good amnesia.

The disadvantages are:
- no clinically useful analgesia
- respiratory depression
- occasional disinhibition effects
- occurrence of sexual fantasies (rare)
- postoperative supervision for a minimum of eight hours is required
- may be unpredictable in children
- elderly patients are easily oversedated.

An absolute contraindication is allergy to any benzodiazepine (very rare). A degree of caution is needed with the following:
- pregnancy and during breast feeding
- severe psychiatric disease
- alcohol or drug abuse
- impairment of hepatic function
- phobia of needles and injections
- poor veins
- domestic responsibilities (e.g. care of children, elderly people)
- doubts about the ability to provide a suitable escort.

Method of administration
The following description of the administration of intravenous midazolam (10 mg/5 ml) is appropriate for most fit and healthy adult patients between 16 and 65 years of age. Even within this age group, variation in the response to sedation is common. Patients outside this age range will be discussed later.

The dental chair should be adjusted to the supine position and the patient made comfortable. Inducing sedation in this position reduces the risk of a vasovagal attack. Monitoring must be established before the patient is sedated to establish baseline readings. Pulse oximetry is mandatory. Continuous blood pressure (BP) and ECG monitoring are not routinely used. However, such monitoring may be advisable for unfit patients. If supplemental oxygen is indicated this is the time to apply the nasal oxygen cannulae and turn on the oxygen (2l/min is sufficient).

Venepuncture

A suitable vein must then be found (see Chapter 2). The most commonly used veins are the metacarpal veins on the dorsum of the hand and the superficial veins of the antecubital fossa; however, any large peripheral vein may be used. In patients with poor veins in the upper limbs, it is often possible

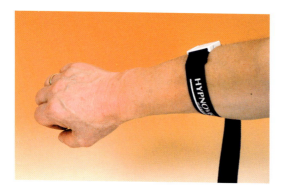

Fig 6-8 Tourniquet.

to use the long saphenous vein in the ankle region or even the small veins on the flexor surface of the wrist. An indwelling cannula should be used for all but exceptional cases. In order to make the veins more prominent the venous return from the limb must be occluded by means of either a carefully placed tourniquet or by having the dental nurse apply firm (but not too firm) pressure around the circumference of the arm (Figs 6-8 and 6-9). The limb must be below the level of the heart to increase venous pooling. Gentle tapping over the selected vein causes local vasodilatation which helps to make the vein visible. The skin may be cleansed with a suitable antiseptic wipe (unless a topical local anaesthetic cream has been used) and the most readily visible and/or palpable vein selected for venepuncture.

The cannula is then inserted into the vein. The angle of approach to the skin surface is important and should be between 20° and 40°. The bevel of the needle should be uppermost. The vein must be stabilised and the skin punctured gently but quickly. The appearance of blood within the chamber of the cannula (flashback) confirms correct placement (Fig 6-10). At this point, the stylet of the cannula is withdrawn and discarded safely (Fig 6-11). Aspiration will confirm the correct siting of the cannula which should then be secured. It is important to remove the tourniquet or ask the assistant to release their grip once venepuncture has been demonstrated to be successful.

Venepuncture, like the administration of an effective inferior dental block, is a simple clinical skill which has to be acquired. Everyone who carries out venepuncture regularly has failures, so do not be discouraged! Some patients have very difficult veins and attend prepared for multiple attempts, having had many similar experiences in the past. A good flow of supportive talk is

Fig 6-9 Nurse applying pressure.

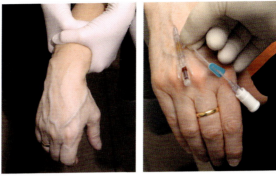

Fig 6-10 Flashback (a positive sign).

Fig 6-11 Appearance of blood in Y-Can line.

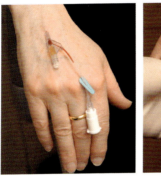
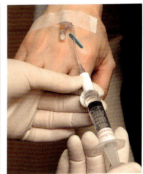

Fig 6-12 Injection of midazolam.

required during the procedure. Advice on performing venepuncture under difficult circumstances is given in Chapter 7.

Midazolam Administration

The prepared drug (10 mg in 5 ml drawn into a 5 ml syringe) is attached to the injection port of the cannula and injected slowly according to the regimen described below (Fig 6-12). The patient should be warned of a cold sensation at the needle site and as the drug tracks up the arm. Provided the sedationist is sure that the needle is correctly sited, the patient should be reassured that this sensation will pass within a short period of time. The injection must be stopped immediately if pain is felt radiating down the limb as this indicates an arterial injection. A complete or partial extravascular injection is usually accompanied by pain and swelling at the site of the injection. In this case the venepuncture must be repeated, preferably in another limb.

Titration Regimen:

1. 2 mg (1 ml) is injected over 30 seconds.
2. Pause for 90 seconds.
3. Further increments of 1 mg (0.5 ml) are administered every 30 seconds until sedation is judged to be adequate.
4. Talk to the patient and watch for any adverse responses, in particular respiratory depression.

The correct dose has been given when there is a slowed response to command, slurring of speech and the patient looks relaxed. Drooping of the eyelids (ptosis), also known as Verrill's sign, is NOT a reliable sign of effective midazolam sedation. Another method of assessing the depth of sedation is to ask the patient to close the eyes and then to try to touch the tip of the nose with the index finger of the limb which has not been cannulated. Inability to demonstrate the appropriate level of coordination is taken to indicate that the patient is adequately sedated.

Patients over the age of 65 years of age usually require much smaller doses of midazolam. A suggested administration regimen for these patients is:
1. 1 mg is injected over 30 seconds.
2. Pause for four minutes.
3. Additional 0.5 mg increments are given every two minutes until sedation is adequate.
Patients in this age group often need only as little as 2 mg of midazolam to provide satisfactory sedation for up to an hour.

If intraoral topical anaesthesia is to be used this should be applied during induction so that local anaesthesia injections can be given as soon as sedation is effective. Dental treatment must be started as quickly as possible to take full advantage of the available working time. Approximately 30 minutes of sedation time is usually available, but this varies from patient to patient. Time should not be wasted. It is acceptable to top up sedation from time to time if the procedure is prolonged but this is rarely necessary during the first 30 minutes. Many routine dental procedures can be completed in this time. If additional increments of midazolam are necessary, 1 mg or 2 mg is usually adequate (less in the elderly). It is important to be aware that topping up rarely achieves the same depth of sedation as that seen immediately following induction. Topping up is unlikely to be successful if the initial level of sedation was inadequate. Under these circumstances, it is better to abandon the procedure and arrange another appointment.

Monitoring the Sedated Patient

The dental team must be constantly aware of the patient's breathing (rate and depth), level of consciousness, airway patency, adequacy of sedation and any changes in skin colour. The use of a pulse oximeter is mandatory. Periodic estimation of heart rate and arterial blood pressure may also be advisable for some patients.

Respiratory rate is quite variable (12–20 breaths per minute in adults) but this is nearly always reduced during sedation and must, therefore, be monitored closely. The depth of breathing is also reduced. Apnoea may occur with an overdose or idiosyncratic response to midazolam. Very shallow ventilation (less than dead space volume) is effectively no ventilation and should be managed as apnoea. This is life threatening if recognition and management are not swift and effective. With intravenous sedation, some degree of respiratory depression is probably present in all patients. Most of the problems associated with inadequate breathing occur in the immediate post-induction period.

Pulse oximetry measures the patient's arterial oxygen saturation and pulse rate from a probe which is attached to the finger or ear lobe. The pulse oximeter detects changes in the patient's oxygen supply, oxygen uptake by the lungs and the delivery of oxygen to the tissues via the circulation (see Chapter 2). It is, as a consequence, an excellent monitor of both respiratory and cardiovascular function. Correct functioning can be affected by metallic nail varnish, cold fingers, fidgeting (causing displacement of the probe) or very bright light falling on the probe. Oxygen saturations below 90% should be investigated and the cause corrected.

Cardiovascular Monitoring: Bradycardia or tachycardia during sedation should be investigated. The former may be related to hypoxia or vagal stimulation whilst the latter is often the result of painful stimuli or anxiety due to undersedation. Most pulse oximeters have audible and visible alarms which are triggered if the heart rate falls or rises beyond clinically acceptable levels. The alarm limit settings depend, to a certain extent, upon the patient. Normally these are 50 beats/min (bradycardia) and 140 beats/min (tachycardia).

As with respiratory rate, blood pressure varies from individual to individual and in the same person under different circumstances. Small variations from so-called normal values are commonplace. The systolic blood pressure is very often raised in anxious subjects by an invasive clinical procedure. Well-controlled hypertension is not an absolute contraindication to sedation. In fact, many patients with high blood pressure are better treated under sedation. For elective intravenous sedation cases, patients with a diastolic blood pressure in excess of 110 mmHg should be investigated before sedation is given.

Recovery and Discharge

At the end of the procedure, the patient should remain under the direct supervision of a suitably trained member of the dental team. Depending on the practice design and facilities, the patient may either be allowed to recover in the dental chair or be moved to a suitably equipped and staffed recovery area. Patients who are unable to walk to the recovery area must continue to be monitored in the dental chair.

Patients must only be discharged by the responsible clinician into the care of a suitable escort who has been given detailed written and verbal instructions covering the next 24 hours (see Chapter 4). No patient should be discharged until sufficiently recovered to stand and walk without assistance. Although most patients will not be fit for discharge until at least one hour following the administration of the last increment of midazolam, there is no fixed time limit, and those responsible for patients during recovery should be discouraged from watching the clock. The patient should rest quietly at home for the remainder of the day. It is important to make the escort aware that the patient should be observed for the first few hours, not simply put to bed out of sight, let alone left "home and alone"!

Reversal of Midazolam Sedation

Flumazenil (Fig 6-13) antagonises the action of midazolam, reversing the sedative (but not amnesic), cardiovascular and respiratory depressant effects (see Chapter 3). Although flumazenil is useful for the management of emergency situations (e.g. benzodiazepine overdose), it may also, for certain patients, make the journey home easier and safer. In, however, most cases this is not necessary. The high cost of this drug makes it unlikely that flumazenil will be used routinely in patients for whom it is neither necessary nor helpful. It must be emphasised that the administration of flumazenil does not reduce the importance of the usual postoperative instructions.

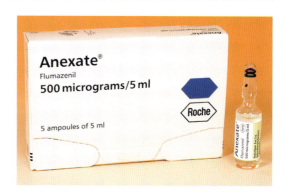

Fig 6-13 Flumazenil ampoule (500 micrograms/5 ml).

Other Sedation Techniques

The following techniques may be helpful for the small proportion of cases where adequate sedation cannot be achieved by intravenous midazolam or inhaled nitrous oxide alone. These must ONLY be used by appropriately trained and experienced practitioners in an appropriate environment.

Intravenous midazolam preceded by an opioid

Individuals who are not adequately sedated using intravenous midazolam alone may sometimes be successfully managed by administering a small bolus of an opioid drug prior to titrating the midazolam. Whilst it is usually preferable to use a single drug, using a combination technique may avoid the need for general anaesthesia.

The opioid selected should ideally have a shorter duration of action than midazolam so as to avoid prolonged recovery. Pethidine, fentanyl, alfentanil and nalbuphine have all been used. For dentistry, nalbuphine has the advantage of not being classified as a controlled drug, which makes its use and storage less complicated. It is administered as follows:

1. Inject 10 mg nalbuphine slowly.
2. Wait for one minute.
3. Titrate midazolam in appropriate increments (as described above).
4. Note that the total dose of midazolam will be probably be considerably less that that required if no opioid is given.

All opioid drugs have the potential to cause dangerous respiratory depression necessitating prompt and effective management from the dental team. The opioid antagonistic, naloxone, must be available (Fig 6-14). Nausea and vomiting are common side effects of these drugs.

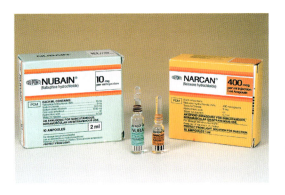

Fig 6-14 Nalbuphine (10 mg/ml) and naloxone (400 micrograms/ml).

Intravenous propofol by operator–controlled infusion

Propofol is a potent short-acting intravenous anaesthetic agent. In sub-anaesthetic concentrations it is a reliable and safe drug for intravenous seda-tion with a considerably shorter distribution half-life than midazolam (see Chapter 3). In comparison with midazolam, recovery is rapid and patients report feeling clear-headed more quickly. Amnesia is often less profound. Propofol confers a greater degree of anxiolysis than sedation and patients appear less "knocked out" than with midazolam. When administered by continuous infusion, propofol is more controllable than titrated midazolam and the depth of sedation may be varied during the procedure (Fig 6-15). It is particularly useful both for very short cases and for lengthy procedures. There are few contraindications to propofol, but it should be avoided if there is known or suspected allergy to any of its components and in patients with epilepsy. Propofol is not licensed for paediatric sedation. Propofol infusion techniques are NOT suitable for use by an operator–sedationist. The tech-nique may only be used by a second practitioner who has received specific training and is experienced.

An example of a method for the administration of propofol sedation is:
1. 30 mg (3 ml) of propofol is given by slow manual injection.
2. An infusion is then started using a syringe pump at an initial rate of 300 mg (30 ml) per hour.
3. Sedation usually occurs within one to two minutes.
4. The infusion rate may need to be adjusted during long procedures.

Particular care is needed with procedures lasting longer than 30 minutes to avoid too deep a level of sedation. Careful clinical monitoring and pulse oximetry are mandatory. Although respiratory depression may occur, it

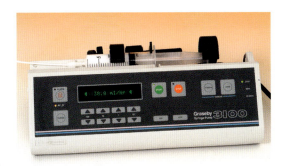

Fig 6-15 Propofol administered by infusion.

appears to be less marked than is the case with midazolam. As with all dental sedation techniques, the use of appropriate local analgesia is essential.
The procedure for recovery is similar to that for midazolam. The criteria for
discharge and instructions for aftercare suggested for midazolam should be
observed.

Intravenous sedation by patient-controlled infusion
Both midazolam and propofol have been used successfully in patient-controlled sedation (PCS) systems. An infusion pump with a demand system
allows the patient to control the depth of sedation. Overdosage is prevented
by a time-based "lockout". In addition to making the patient feel more in
control, PCS may optimise the level of sedation and thus reduce the incidence of both under- and oversedation.

Oral sedation with benzodiazepines
Oral benzodiazepines may be useful in cases in which the patient is anxious
about venepuncture or where cannulation is impossible due to lack of cooperation – for example, in the case of patients with certain physical or learning disabilities.

The sedation produced may be sufficient for simple dental procedures to be
carried out. Alternatively, it may be employed to facilitate cannulation for
intravenous sedation. The most commonly used drugs are temazepam (adult
dose: 30 mg) or midazolam (adult dose: 20 mg).

Temazepam is best administered as a proprietary oral syrup, which is reasonably palatable, rather than as tablets, which may be difficult to swallow. The
time to peak effect is variable. Typically, adequate sedation occurs approxi-

mately 30–45 minutes following ingestion of the drug. Sedation must be administered in the dental surgery under the supervision of the dentist. Temazepam 30 mg may be expected to produce a similar depth of sedation as is usually achieved with a correctly titrated dose of intravenous midazolam.

There is currently no readily available proprietary preparation of midazolam for oral use in the United Kingdom. The intravenous preparation (either 10 mg/2 ml or 10 mg/5 ml) is, however, suitable for oral administration. Midazolam has a bitter taste and should be added to a strong tasting fruit juice to improve its palatability. The time to peak effect is less variable than with temazepam. Using midazolam, sedation usually occurs approximately 10–20 minutes following ingestion of the drug. As with temazepam, sedation must be administered in the dental surgery under supervision of the dentist.

The management of patients who have received oral temazepam or midazolam is very similar to that for those who have received intravenous midazolam. As the depth of sedation is similar, clinical monitoring and the use of a pulse oximeter are mandatory and the discharge criteria are identical.

Although midazolam is used for conscious sedation in dentistry, it does not have a UK product licence for oral administration. However, the oral route is commonly used in other areas of sedation practice – for example, accident and emergency medicine. There is also a large body of published evidence relating to its safety and efficacy.

It is important to appreciate that the apparent simplicity of oral sedation belies the potential for undesirable effects in addition to the desired sedative effect. In particular, the risk of respiratory depression is every bit as great with oral sedation as it is with intravenous midazolam. If possible, once sedation is established, a cannula should be inserted to enable the administration of flumazenil in the event of problems.

Intranasal sedation using midazolam

Midazolam may also be administered intranasally. As with oral administration, this application is currently unlicensed. In adults, 10 mg of the 10 mg/2 ml concentration is usually sufficient and is surprisingly well tolerated by patients. Intranasal midazolam is rapidly absorbed through the nasal mucosa directly into the circulation and therefore the peak effect occurs sooner than with the oral route. Patient monitoring and discharge criteria are identical to those for intravenous sedation with midazolam. This technique finds particular application in patients with disabilities who are unable to cooperate sufficiently for more conventional routes of administration to be successful. As with oral sedation, the potential for adverse effects must be considered carefully. Neither of these techniques allows accurate titration of midazolam against the patient's response. With such fixed-dose techniques there is always a risk of unpredicted under- or oversedation.

Conclusions

- Inhalational sedation (Relative Analgesia) and intravenous sedation with midazolam are the most widely used techniques.
- Knowledge of alternative drugs and routes of administration may occasionally be helpful in specialist environments.
- The simplest technique is usually the most appropriate.

Further Reading

Health and Safety Executive. Occupational Exposure Limits. London: HMSO, 1998.

Roberts GJ. Inhalation sedation (relative analgesia) with oxygen/nitrous oxide gas mixtures. 1. Principles. Dent Update 1990;17:139–146.

Roberts GJ. Inhalation sedation (relative analgesia) with oxygen/nitrous oxide gas mixtures. 2. Practical techniques. Dent Update 1990;17:190–196.

Skelly AM. Sedation in dental practice. Dent Update 1992;19:61–67.

Chapter 7

Complications: Avoidance and Management

Aim

The aim of this chapter is to describe the management of sedation-related problems and complications.

Outcome

After reading this chapter you should be able to recognise and manage common complications associated with the administration of conscious sedation in general dental practice and other primary care settings.

Introduction

Serious complications associated with carefully administered conscious sedation are rare. Minor problems are more common. Fortunately, most minor problems are easily managed by a well-prepared dental team. Careful case selection, based on a detailed medical, dental and social history, will often allow the dental team to anticipate potential difficulties and take appropriate action. Prevention is always preferable to treatment.

Although complications may arise from the use of any sedation technique, it is a widely held misconception that intravenous sedation offers the greatest potential for difficulties. This chapter will consider only those complications which may arise from intravenous sedation using midazolam and inhalational sedation using nitrous oxide and oxygen. The reader is referred to the descriptions of alternative drugs in Chapter 6 for brief comments on the possible difficulties associated with these techniques.

Complications of Sedation and their Management

Respiratory depression

The most serious potential complication associated with intravenous sedation using midazolam is respiratory depression. The mechanisms for this are described in detail in Chapter 2. Put simply, the patient "forgets to breathe" and the normal physiological corrective mechanisms fail to respond.

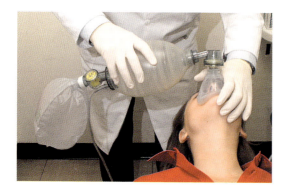

Fig 7-1 Intermittent positive pressure ventilation.

It is important to understand that all patients who receive intravenous midazolam experience some reduction in both the rate and the depth of breathing. This is sometimes apparent clinically (chest movement is visibly reduced) but not always. The effect is usually most pronounced during the first 10 minutes or so of sedation. It is sometimes seen much later, particularly when there is a lull in clinical activity. The difficulty in recognising mild or even moderate respiratory depression underlines the necessity for continuous pulse oximetry in addition to careful clinical monitoring.

Management of midazolam–induced respiratory depression involves the following steps:
• Ask the patient to take several deep breaths.

In the majority of cases, this will resolve the problem; BUT if this fails:
• Open the airway (head tilt/chin lift or jaw thrust) and perform intermittent positive pressure ventilation using a ventilating bag, preferably with an oxygen supply attached (Fig 7-1).

IF this fails:
• Administer flumazenil (500 micrograms by slow intravenous injection). Continue to ventilate and encourage breathing.

Note that it is VERY rarely necessary to do anything more than encourage breathing.

Airway obstruction
Obstruction of the airway may occur during any form of sedation. Patients who have received intravenous drugs are probably less likely to notice and

to complain of breathing problems. Excessive downward pressure without adequate support of the mandible during the extraction of molar teeth is a common cause, the management of which is obvious. Accumulation of water and dental debris in the oropharynx can also be a problem. This is easily managed by the use of properly positioned high-volume suction. Carrying out restorative procedures under rubber dam is a most effective way of minimising this difficulty. In the event of respiratory problems, the rubber dam must be removed immediately.

Hypotension

All intravenous sedation drugs tend to cause a decrease in the systemic arterial blood pressure. This is partly due to reduced sympathetic activity and direct depression of the brain's cardiac control centres. Unlike respiratory depression, the fall in blood pressure is usually self-limiting and, as such, requires no active treatment. A patient with a naturally low arterial blood pressure should be moved slowly from the supine position to the sitting position to reduce the possibility of postural hypotension. A patient with a very low resting blood pressure may benefit from intermittent blood pressure monitoring.

Problems with Venepuncture

Intravenous cannulation is easily learned but, like many clinical skills, proficiency takes time and minor problems are commonplace, particularly during the early days. The similarity with learning to administer an effective inferior dental block is perhaps helpful – initial anxiety associated with a high failure rate is soon followed by an improved rate of success and confidence. With more experience, this matures into a more realistic approach which enables the confident management of occasional failure.

The most common problems associated with venepuncture are:
• failure to find a suitable vein
• difficulty in siting the cannula in the lumen of the vein
• failure to obtain flashback
• painful, extravascular injection
• bruising following removal of the cannula.

Whilst most patients have a variety of medium-sized and visible veins in either the antecubital fossa or on the dorsum of the hand, a few patients appear to have been born without a venous system. Anxiety, cold weather and a history of intravenous drug abuse can also make finding a suitable vein extremely difficult.

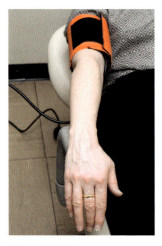

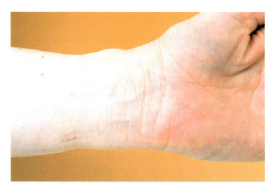

Fig 7-2 Sphygmomanometer used to aid venepuncture.

Fig 7-3 Veins on the flexor surface of wrist.

The following tips and tricks may be helpful:
- Ask the patient to wear gloves and warm clothing on the way to the practice.
- Place patient's hands in warm water.
- Use a sphygmomanometer cuff inflated to a pressure somewhere between the patient's systolic and diastolic blood pressure (Fig 7-2).
- Ensure that the limb is below the level of the heart.
- Gently stimulate (tap) over the chosen site.
- Shine the dental light across the hand or antecubital fossa.
- Consider alternative sites, e.g. flexor surface of the wrist (Fig 7-3).
- Ask the patient if they know where a suitable vein may be found.
- Avoid offering intravenous sedation to individuals with poor veins.

Difficulty in inserting a cannula into the chosen vein is often related to poor preparation or faulty technique. A common problem is entering the wall of the vein rather than the lumen. The cannula appears to be in the vein but there is no flashback. This can sometimes be corrected by a quick realignment of the cannula, but this procedure is difficult with the relatively small gauge cannulae used for dental sedation. It is often better to remove the cannula completely and try another site on another limb. An immediate further attempt at venepuncture on the same arm or hand will cause bleeding and bruising.

Although flashback strongly suggests that the cannula is correctly sited this is not always the case. The first increment of the intravenous drug should always be administered slowly whilst observing the area of skin overlying the tip of the cannula. Similarly, absence of flashback does not always indicate failure – a small quantity of saline may be injected prior to administering the sedative drug to confirm that the cannula is correctly sited.

Extravascular injection of midazolam is usually uncomfortable. If this occurs the cannula must be repositioned. Intra-arterial injections are rare, even when the medial aspect of the antecubital fossa is used. Intra-arterial injections cause pain which runs down the arm. If this is suspected, the injection must be stopped and the cannula resited, as above. Although painful, intra-arterial midazolam is unlikely to cause long-term sequelae.

A small amount of bruising is common following any intravenous injection. This can be minimised by maintaining firm pressure over the puncture site whilst keeping the limb raised above the level of the heart.

Hiccups
A small number of patients experience hiccups following intravenous sedation with midazolam. Unlike normal bouts of hiccups, which usually persist for less than 30 minutes, hiccups associated with intravenous sedation may last for hours or even overnight. Whilst there is clearly no risk involved, the condition may cause considerable distress.

Most cases of prolonged hiccups appear to be associated with either excessive midazolam or rapid injection (or both). It may, therefore, be prudent to administer the drug more slowly in patients who are known to be susceptible. There is no tried and tested treatment for midazolam-induced hiccups. An explanation and reassurance should be given to both the patient and their escort. Any of the well-known folk remedies may be worth a try.

Allergy
Allergy to all benzodiazepines is rare. Midazolam may be regarded as a very safe drug for intravenous sedation. In the unlikely event of an anaphylactic reaction, the treatment should include oxygen, epinephrine, calling for assistance, etc. Flumazenil must NOT be administered. Allergic reactions to nitrous oxide are unheard of.

Nausea and vomiting
Many anxious dental patients feel sick at the thought of a visit to the sur-

gery. There are also a great many patients who have suffered nausea or vomiting associated with the administration of general anaesthesia, in particular dental general anaesthesia. Patients may, therefore, attend for dental treatment under sedation expecting either to feel or to be sick. Such patients should be reassured that neither midazolam nor nitrous oxide is likely to cause nausea or vomiting – a little reassurance goes a long way. Patients who regularly vomit following sedation may benefit from the administration of an antiemetic drug (e.g. metoclopramide) during induction.

Prolonged recovery

Recovery from nitrous oxide sedation normally take place within a matter of minutes. Recovery from intravenous midazolam is more variable due to variability in redistribution of the drug from the receptor sites (short–term recovery) followed by metabolism and excretion (long–term recovery). Some groups of patients (particularly those taking or using CNS depressant drugs) have notoriously unpredictable recovery times. For the majority of these patients, management simply involves patience and careful monitoring. Flumazenil may be helpful, but should not normally be used when the patient has psychiatric or medical conditions which involve treatment with potent central nervous system depressants or stimulants, in particular benzodiazepines. An exception to this rule may be made in the case of a patient with prolonged recovery and profound respiratory depression that cannot be managed by simple methods.

Failure of sedation

Sedation techniques do not always work as well as the dentist and the patient might like. Early recognition of impending failure is important to avoid starting a dental procedure which it may not be possible to complete. "Quit while you are ahead" is an excellent axiom. The most common reasons for failed sedation, and some possible solutions, are discussed in Chapter 8. An open and honest discussion with the patient and their escort will reduce the disappointment of a failed sedation session.

Paradoxical effects

Intravenous sedation sometimes results in a paradoxical effect. The patient becomes more rather than less anxious and treatment may be impossible. This is particularly common in children and adolescents. The administration of more midazolam often makes matters worse and the effects of flumazenil are unpredictable. The best approach is to abandon treatment and allow the patient to rest quietly. Orally administered midazolam may be an alternative for such patients.

98

Disinhibition

Many patients show signs of mild disinhibition when sedated with midazolam. Such patients may have bouts of giggling, crying, talkativeness or even panic attacks that may seriously interfere with dental treatment. Firm management by the dental team may restore calm and tranquillity but further bouts can occur. Aggressive and abusive behaviour is probably another manifestation of disinhibition. In such cases, it is up to the dental team to draw the line between acceptable and unacceptable behaviour. In mitigation, most abusive patients are probably unaware of their bad behaviour under sedation.

Oversedation

A small amount of oversedation with intravenous midazolam is not usually a serious problem. The most common effect is poor patient cooperation. The patient often refuses to open the mouth and so the start of treatment is delayed. Waiting a few minutes usually resolves the difficulty. Gross oversedation using midazolam may cause profound respiratory depression or even apnoea requiring prompt and effective management.

Mild oversedation with nitrous oxide is often more troublesome as the patient may feel panicky and even pull the nasal mask off their face. Oversedation of young children is particularly undesirable. The unpleasant side effects may make further treatment under inhalational sedation impossible. Severe oversedation with nitrous oxide may produce light anaesthesia with associated limb and eye movements.

Undersedation

Whilst taking every care to avoid oversedation, it is important to ensure that the patient is adequately sedated. Undersedation is pointless and may lead to increased dental phobia. Failing to provide an adequate depth of sedation is a common failure of the inexperienced sedationist who believes, incorrectly, that this is associated with an increased level of safety. Few dentists would intentionally inject insufficient local anaesthesic for a potentially painful dental procedure.

Sexual fantasies

Much has been written about the occurrence of sexual fantasies in patients receiving intravenous sedation using midazolam. The extent of the problem is unknown. The best advice which can be offered is to ensure that no sedated (or recovering) patient is ever left alone with only one member of the dental team.

Record Keeping

In addition to the normal records relating to the administration of sedation and dental treatment, the dentist should make detailed notes relating to any problem which occurs during sedation. This is not only for medicolegal reasons, but also to assist in the appropriate management of the patient on subsequent occasions.

Conclusions

- Serious complications are rare with conscious sedation.
- Midazolam-induced respiratory depression requires prompt diagnosis and effective management.
- Venepuncture is sometimes difficult.
- Good record keeping is essential.

Useful Website

Resuscitation Council (UK): www.resus.org.uk.

Chapter 8
Sedation in Special Circumstances

Aim

The aim of this chapter is to describe the impact of medical conditions on sedation in dental practice and to discuss the recognition and management of failed sedation.

Outcome

After reading this chapter you should have an understanding of the medical conditions for which sedation is indicated and contraindicated in general dental practice and other primary dental care settings.

Introduction

Whilst simple dental sedation techniques are appropriate, safe and successful for the majority of fit and cooperative patients, it is important to recognise that some individuals (medically compromised patients, special care patients, paediatric patients) present special problems. This may require a more flexible approach involving management tailored to the particular needs of the individual. Sedation in these circumstances is usually best provided in a specialist centre by practitioners with appropriate training and experience.

Medically Compromised Patients

Not all medical conditions compromise the dental care of patients, but all have an impact on their daily lives. Only those common disorders which might influence sedation will be discussed. The most important of these are those relating to the cardiovascular and respiratory systems, although some musculoskeletal disorders are also significant. It is important to appreciate that, in many cases, it is positively helpful to prescribe sedation, whereas, in others, sedation techniques may require modification. The administration of supplemental oxygen may be indicated in the management of many of these patients.

Conditions in which sedation is beneficial

Sedation is almost certainly beneficial in conditions such as angina, hypertension, asthma, epilepsy and movement disorders.

Angina: Angina may be provoked by anxiety or stress before, during and even after a dental procedure. This often causes tachycardia and increases the work of the heart which may result in the characteristic ischaemic pain of angina. In addition to careful and sensitive patient management, including effective local anaesthesia, the provision of sedation further protects the patient from the effects of stress and so significantly reduces the likelihood of an angina attack.

When considering whether to sedate a patient who suffers from angina in a primary care setting, it is important to differentiate between controlled (stable) angina and uncontrolled (unstable) angina. The former is not usually a contraindication to the use of conscious sedation whereas patients with unstable angina should only be treated in specialist centres.

The emergency management of an angina attack during sedation is no different from that provided for a patient being treated under local anaesthesia alone. It is sometimes appropriate to ask the patient to use their routine rescue medication – for example, glyceryl trinitrate, immediately before the start of treatment (Fig 8-1).

Hypertension: Most patients with diagnosed high blood pressure take medication but control may not always be optimal. There are also many patients with hypertension who are undiagnosed and so blood pressure measurement at the assessment visit is essential. It is generally accepted that a persistent

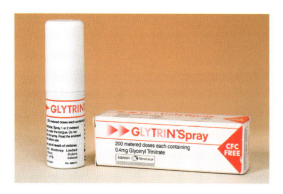

Fig 8-1   Glyceryl trinitrate spray.

diastolic blood pressure in excess of 110 mmHg represents a contraindication to the use of sedation in other than a specialist centre. Remember that blood pressure tends to increase with age and should be reassessed periodically.

Anxiety brought on by the prospect of dental treatment can cause an increase in heart rate and elevation of blood pressure in hypertensive patients. Sedation modifies these responses and protects the patient against sudden changes in blood pressure which can, in extreme cases, precipitate more serious cardiovascular events – for example, cerebrovascular accidents (CVA) or angina. Note that patients with low blood pressure are likely to suffer postural hypotension following sedation.

Asthma: Asthma appears to be an increasing problem within the population at large. Well-controlled asthma is not a contraindication to the use of sedation. Where asthma is poorly controlled, even with medication (brittle asthma), great care must be exercised. Sedation may be helpful, but a detailed assessment of the patient on each day of treatment is essential as asthma is notoriously labile.

Emergency management of an asthma attack during sedation is similar to that necessary for a patient being treated under local anaesthesia. But increased attention must be paid to respiratory function, in particular, if a respiratory depressant drug, such as midazolam, is in use. Rescue treatment usually involves oxygen therapy, inhaling salbutamol (Fig 8-2) and possibly steroids and attention to the positioning of the patient (Fig 8-3). As with angina, it is sometimes appropriate to ask the patient to use their routine res-

Fig 8-2 Salbutamol inhaler.   **Fig 8-3** Asthma: patient positioned to aid breathing.

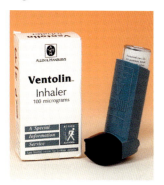

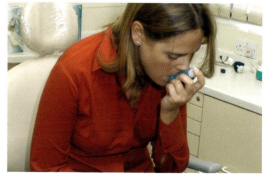

cue medication immediately prior to treatment. Severe (brittle) asthmatics are at risk and must be managed by a specialist team.

Epilepsy: Grand mal epilepsy is often associated with other neurological disorders and in syndromes associated with learning disability. In assessing the advisability of using sedation in a person with epilepsy, the frequency of seizures is probably the most useful index of the severity of the condition. Patients with well-controlled epilepsy usually present few problems, whereas the uncontrolled or poorly controlled patient must be referred for specialist care.

Antiepileptic drugs all depress the central nervous system. As such, they may interact with central nervous system depressant sedation agents. The outcome may be either tolerance to, or potentiation of the sedative effect. Practically speaking, this often produces unpredictable over- or undersedation and a shortened period of effective anxiolysis. Nonetheless, intravenous midazolam usually provides excellent sedation and also reduces the risk of stress-induced seizures.

Emergency supportive management of a patient who fits under sedation is no different from normal. Flumazenil should not be used unless there is also profound respiratory depression or apnoea which cannot be treated with intermittent positive pressure ventilation with oxygen.

Movement disorders: In patients with uncontrolled movements or spasticity, intravenous benzodiazepine sedation will often reduce or suppress excess activity, making treatment easier for both the dentist and the patient.

Conditions where the technique might require modification
Modification of the sedation technique might be required in conditions such as myocardial infarction, heart failure, anaemia, chronic obstructive pulmonary disease, diabetes mellitus and pregnancy.

Myocardial infarction: A patient who has had a myocardial infarct should not receive elective dental treatment under intravenous sedation until at least six months after the heart attack. Nitrous oxide may provide a suitable alternative. A patient whose cardiac condition remains unstable must only be sedated by an appropriately experienced sedationist. Supplemental oxygen through nasal cannulae is mandatory in such cases (Fig 8-4).

Heart failure: This may be due to right or left ventricular failure. In either case, there may be respiratory distress if the patient is treated in the supine position. Careful questioning of the patient about their sleeping position may serve as a guide for positioning the dental chair. A compromise must be made between the aggravation of dyspnoea and postural hypotension. Liver perfusion may be reduced and drug metabolism therefore delayed. This could result in prolonged recovery from those sedative drugs which undergo metabolism in the liver – for example, midazolam.

Anaemia: Individuals with anaemia are at increased risk of hypoxia because of reduction in oxygen carrying haemoglobin. A patient with suspected anaemia should be investigated by their general medical practitioner before sedation is offered. Pulse oximetry may be

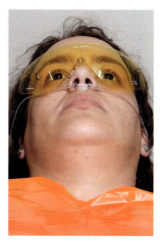

Fig 8-4 Supplemental oxygen via nasal cannulae.

unreliable and cyanosis appears later in patients with anaemia, so careful monitoring of respiration and prompt intervention are essential.

Chronic obstructive pulmonary disease (COPD): As with heart failure, posture in the dental chair may have to be compromised to allow comfortable breathing. Many patients with COPD have a productive cough and a sensitive upper airway, causing frequent coughing and spluttering which may be exacerbated by dental procedures. Frequent paroxysmal coughing disrupts the sedative effect and makes good quality dentistry difficult. It may be better to defer treatment during, or immediately following, an acute upper respiratory tract infection in such patients.

Patients with COPD – in particular those who smoke – often present with a low baseline oxygen saturation. Supplemental oxygen should be started before the induction of sedation in these cases. Patients with very severe bronchitis who may have a hypoxic respiratory drive should not be sedated with benzodiazepines or other respiratory depressant agents.

Diabetes mellitus: A patient with well-controlled diabetes presents few problems as long as they continue their usual medication and are not asked to fast before treatment. As discussed elsewhere (Chapter 9), there is no need for patients to abstain from either food or non-alcoholic drinks on the day

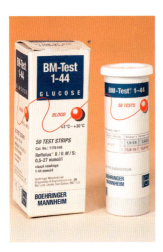

of treatment under conscious sedation. Poorly controlled diabetes presents a risk of hypoglycaemia being masked by post-sedation drowsiness. For this reason, a patient whose diabetes is not well controlled should be referred for further medical assessment and treatment before being offered sedation.

In an emergency, chairside measurement of blood sugar is possible using a variety of simple techniques (Fig 8-5). The results require careful interpretation and immediate medical advice should be obtained – in particular, if consciousness is lost.

Fig 8-5 BM-Test for chairside blood glucose estimation.

Pregnancy: There is no sedation drug which is guaranteed to be safe during pregnancy.

As far as possible the use of sedation should be avoided in the first trimester. If dental treatment cannot be deferred, nitrous oxide is probably preferable to midazolam. In later pregnancy, the use of nitrous oxide is generally considered to be safe.

Mothers who are breast feeding should be warned that some sedative drugs – for example, midazolam – are secreted in breast milk and can produce a degree of sedation in their infant. This may not always be perceived as an unwelcome side effect.

Conditions where caution is required
Caution is required, and referral should be considered, for conditions such as advanced cardiorespiratory disease, active liver disease, severe psychological/psychiatric disease, drug and/or alcohol abuse and obesity.

Advanced cardiorespiratory disease: Patients who are breathless at rest or after minimal exertion should not be considered for treatment under conscious sedation anywhere other than a specialist centre.

Active liver disease: If there is active liver disease, known liver failure, or impairment of liver function, drug effects may be magnified due to changes in plasma protein concentrations. Small doses produce exaggerated effects due to increased levels of free drug. Metabolism may be very slow and recovery dangerously prolonged. Additionally, these patients often present bleeding and healing problems which may affect treatment. Assessment and treatment by a specialist is essential.

Severe psychological illness: Individuals with unpredictable behaviour present management problems. They may also react abnormally to sedative drugs due to concurrent psychoactive medication. The onset and precise effects of sedatives may be altered and distorted. Recovery and post-sedation behaviour are unpredictable. The effect of flumazenil is often idiosyncratic. The effectiveness of sedation may vary widely on different occasions, possibly due to changes in medication and the course of the underlying illness. The patient's social circumstances may be such that they cannot provide a reliable escort.

Drug and alcohol abuse: These conditions are often associated with psychiatric disease. Even where this is not the case, the impact of drugs and alcohol may result in a variety of difficulties. Liver failure and chronic viral infections are common. Many intravenous drug users have very poor veins which may make venepuncture in conventional and acceptable sites difficult. Some also develop a morbid fear of needles and injections. It is not uncommon for patients to self-administer a "pre-med" of their favourite agent prior to attending to reduce their anxiety and to increase the sedative effects of the prescribed conscious sedation agent. Escorts are often recruited from acquaintances who may be no more responsible than the patient. This may make inpatient care the only safe option.

Obesity: Individuals with a body mass index (BMI) greater than 25 may not be suitable for treatment under conscious sedation in the dental surgery. Obese patients often have difficult veins. In the event of a collapse, there may be airway management and patient handling problems. Some dental chairs may become unstable or fail to operate correctly if their maximum load is exceeded. Careful assessment, including an estimation of the BMI, is indicated for overweight patients. The BMI is calculated by dividing the patient's weight (kilograms) by the square of the height (metres^2).

Concurrent medication: Medicines can alert the sedationist to undisclosed disease and raise the possibility of potential drug interactions. Some medicines interact with, or potentiate the action of, sedative drugs and may also alter recovery time. Other drugs share metabolic pathways with benzodiazepines and can delay recovery. Drugs with potential interactions include antidepressants, other benzodiazepines, antihistamines, opioid analgesics, alcohol, H2 receptor antagonists, protease inhibitors and erythromycin. None of these drugs represents an absolute contraindication to the use of sedation.

Medical Risk Assessment

In adult patients, the ASA fitness scale is a good guide (see Chapter 4). It is wise to be cautious with patients who suffer from two or more relevant illnesses, particularly if they are taking multiple drugs. Although it may be possible to classify patients such as ASA II, in these situations, it may be better to consider the patients as ASA III. If there is any doubt, the patient should be referred for specialist advice and treatment. For example, an elderly patient with one controlled illness (e.g. angina) is probably suitable for treatment in general practice. The presence of a second known condition (e.g. type 1 diabetes) suggests referral, bearing in mind that further disease processes may also be present but undiagnosed.

Smoking can reduce respiratory efficiency to the extent that hypoxia may be seen during intravenous sedation. Supplemental oxygen should be used in smokers whose baseline oxygen saturation is below 94% before induction of sedation. Coughing and spluttering during sedation is common and disruptive.

Special Care Patients

The provision of dental care for people with learning or physical disabilities may not be possible using local anaesthesia and standard sedation techniques. This may be as a result of difficulties in communication between the patient and the dental team, or a physical inability to cooperate, as is sometimes the case in individuals with uncontrolled movements. In the past, many of these patients were managed using general anaesthesia. Whilst this may remain appropriate and necessary for a number of patients, the use of novel sedation techniques has reduced this need and increased the range and quality of care that can be provided. Many patients requiring special care dentistry have concomitant medical problems. These must be assessed when considering the use of sedation.

The simplest and safest sedation technique should be selected for each individual patient. The length and nature of the dental procedure must also be considered. Suitably trained and experienced practitioners often successfully treat people with mild or moderate learning disabilities with oral or inhalation sedation. The patient with severe learning disabilities and challenging behaviour may exhibit resistant or aggressive behaviour and, as a consequence, communication may be extremely difficult. Physical disability may also present more practical problems – for example, transport and positioning in an ordinary dental chair. In addition, uncontrolled movements may also put the patient and dental team at physical risk. For these patients, inhalation sedation is not usually possible and intravenous cannulation may be both difficult and hazardous.

Alternative sedation techniques which have been used successfully in these patients include:
• orally administered midazolam
• intranasal midazolam
• either of the above followed by intravenous midazolam or propofol
• intravenous propofol infusion
• ketamine (with or without intravenous midazolam).

All these techniques require considerable additional training and experience and must only be offered by teams who are both competent and equipped to provide the appropriate sedation technique, clinical care and management of such patients.

Paediatric Patients

In the UK, inhalational sedation using a titrated dose of nitrous oxide in oxygen (Relative Analgesia) as described in Chapter 6 is the only well-tried and tested sedation technique currently recommended for children.

Intravenous sedation with midazolam is often said to be "reliably unpredictable" in patients under 16 years of age and "predictably unreliable" under 12 years of age. For reasons which are not properly understood, some young patients appear to respond differently from adults to intravenously administered benzodiazepines. Some children sedate satisfactorily whilst others become disinhibited, more anxious or even aggressive. Despite a number of recent studies it has not been possible to identify any factor or group of factors which may be used to predict the likelihood of success. Therefore, until more research has been carried out, intravenous midazolam should be considered for children only when other options cannot be used. In any case, these techniques must only be used by experienced sedationists or anaesthetists working in an appropriate environment. The use of flumazenil to manage a young patient with disinhibition following intravenous midazolam is not recommended as the data currently available suggest that the situation is often made worse rather than improved. Of course, if there is profound respiratory depression which cannot be managed by stimulating the patient and, if necessary, using intermittent positive pressure ventilation, flumazenil is indicated (see Chapter 6). Propofol is widely used for adult sedation but it does not have a licence for paediatric sedation in the UK.

Orally administered benzodiazepines (for example, temazepam, midazolam) appear to produce reliable sedation for this age group. The time taken for the drug to act is much less predictable than with intravenous sedation, given differences in the rate of gastric absorption, first-pass metabolism and protein binding. Using temazepam, most patients become sedated somewhere between 30 and 45 minutes following oral administration. Midazolam appears to be the more predictable drug in this respect with a typical time of onset of about 12 minutes. Midazolam does not currently have a UK licence for oral administration, but is licensed in most other parts of the world including mainland Europe and North America. Its widespread use in the UK in dental and medical disciplines has shown this to be a safe, appropriate and effective technique. Orally administered antihistamines have been used for paediatric sedation in medicine for many years, but their use in dentistry has mostly been limited to special care patients. Benzodiazepines may also be administered intranasally and although this technique offers a number of advantages for certain groups – in particular, very young patients, needle phobics and those with disabilities – the route is unlicensed and requires special training and experience.

It is important to remember that oral sedation produces a similar level of sedation to that achieved by intravenous midazolam. As a consequence, the pre- and postoperative instructions to the patient, monitoring and arrangements for discharge are identical to those for intravenous sedation. Oral sedation should not be regarded as a safer or easier option than intravenous sedation. In many ways, it is potentially less safe given the poor predictability of onset, depth of sedation and recovery.

Inhalational sedation using sevoflurane in oxygen (or a mixture of nitrous oxide and oxygen) is currently being researched and it appears to be useful for younger patients. Sevoflurane is a potent volatile anaesthetic agent with a favourable blood gas solubility and a low MAC (see Chapter 3). Induction is rapid and the relatively high potency controlled by a suitably calibrated vaporiser. At present, sevoflurane sedation must be administered only by trained anaesthetists.

Whichever technique is used for paediatric sedation, it is a requirement that practitioners and their teams are experienced in the use of the drug and its route of administration.

Failed Sedation

Recognition

Sedation techniques are not always successful. Failure may occur for a variety of reasons relating to the patient, the operator, or the technique chosen. The more challenging the patient and the more difficult the sedation and dental procedure, the greater the likelihood of failure. No sedationist achieves 100% success with all patients. The most common causes of failure include:
- incorrect patient assessment
- unrealistic expectations (patient or dentist)
- failure to accept that anxiolysis is not oblivion
- poor dental treatment planning
- technique failure (e.g. venepuncture, LA, psychological support)
- missing the IV sedation "window" (e.g. hesitant dentistry)
- "bad sedation day".

Management

As soon as it becomes clear that the chosen sedation technique is not going to allow the intended treatment to be completed to the satisfaction of both patient and dentist, it is advisable to stop and carry out whatever temporary measures are indicated so the patient can be discharged comfortably and safely. Continuing with treatment on a protesting patient is doomed to failure and likely to produce dissatisfaction and even complaints. Additionally, subsequent treatment may be made more difficult as the patient will have lost confidence.

The disappointment of failure can be overcome by adopting an honest, flexible and positive approach. If the patient is still sedated or upset, it is probably better to arrange another appointment for future treatment planning. When discussing this with the patient and the escort, it is important to be reassuring whilst not promising the impossible. If there are appropriate facilities and expertise in the practice, alternative sedation techniques may be considered and the possible advantages outlined. If other techniques cannot be offered, or it is clear that the patient does not wish to return, a referral should be made for treatment under alternative sedation techniques or even general anaesthesia. The alternative techniques (discussed in Chapter 6) include:
- multidrug intravenous sedation (e.g. an opioid and a benzodiazepine)

- propofol infusion
- patient-controlled sedation (midazolam or propofol)
- oral/intranasal benzodiazepines
- volatile agents (e.g. sevoflurane).

Possible cases for referral for general anaesthesia include:
- some medically compromised patients (e.g. severe asthma, proven allergy to all local anaesthetics)
- people with disabilities who cannot be managed with sedation
- paediatric patients (e.g. uncooperative children, extensive treatment)
- failed sedation patients
- adult patients requiring extensive, long or unpleasant treatment.

The successful management of patient groups discussed in this chapter requires considerable investment in training and facilities (see Chapter 9).

Conclusions

- Sedation is beneficial when providing dental treatment for patients with some medical conditions.
- Sedation in dental practice is contraindicated for patients with some medical conditions.
- Sedation sometimes fails.

Further Reading

Boyle C. Sedation for the Special Patient. In: Word of Mouth – Dental Health and Practice 2002. London: British Dental Health Foundation, 2000:161–163.

Manley M, Skelly A, Hamilton A. Dental treatment for people with challenging behaviour: general anaesthesia or sedation? Br Dent J 2000;188:358–360.

Chapter 9
Standards of Good Practice and Medicolegal Considerations

Aim

The aim of this chapter is to review the current UK recommendations relating to conscious sedation.

Outcome

After reading this chapter you should have an understanding of the principles of safe sedation practice as described by the General Dental Council (GDC) and the Department of Health.

Introduction

The practice of conscious sedation in the UK has been the subject of intense medicolegal interest since the publication of the Poswillo Report in 1990. There have been at least twelve original detailed reports, guidelines and recommendations published since Poswillo (Fig 9-1). This is far in excess of

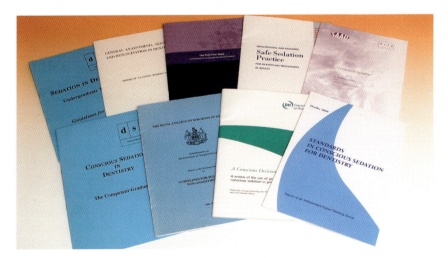

Fig 9-1 The plethora of guidelines for dental sedation.

Table 9-1 Current UK guidelines for sedation in dentistry.

2000	Department of Health	*A Conscious Decision*
2000	Independent Working Group	*Standards in Conscious Sedation*
2001	General Dental Council	*Maintaining Standards*
2001	UK Academy of Medical Royal Colleges	*Safe Sedation Practice*
2003	Department of Health	*Guidelines for Conscious Sedation*

similar guidance for any other area of dental practice or, indeed, for the practice of conscious sedation in medical specialties. Many of these reports have simply reiterated or expanded upon the messages of earlier documents. Given the excellent safety record of conscious sedation for dentistry in the UK, the reader is left to speculate whether this intense scrutiny is necessary or helpful.

The medicolegal guidelines for sedation practice, shown in Table 9-1, are a summary of current UK recommendations available at the time of writing.

There is general recognition that the management of pain and anxiety is of fundamental importance for patients requiring dental care and that conscious sedation is effective and safe. The concept of the operator-sedationist – the practitioner who carries out the dental treatment and also administers the conscious sedation – is fully supported.

The GDC's Current Definition of Conscious Sedation

"A technique in which the use of a drug or drugs produces a state of depression of the central nervous system enabling treatment to be carried out, but during which verbal contact with the patient is maintained throughout the period of sedation. The drugs and techniques used to provide conscious sedation for dental treatment should carry a margin of safety wide enough to render loss of consciousness unlikely."

Note that the definition describes the **state** of conscious sedation, and does not attempt to prescribe **how** it is achieved. It is acknowledged that techniques involving the use of one or more drugs administered via different routes will fulfil this definition.

Training

All members of the dental team providing treatment under conscious sedation must receive appropriate and supervised theoretical, practical and clinical training before undertaking independent practice (Figs 9-2 and 9-3). Theoretical and non-clinical skills training should be completed before clinical training is commenced. This should include the management of sedation-related complications. Supervised hands–on clinical experience must be acquired by practitioners and the members of their dental team for each sedation technique to be used.

Guidance on clinical training for dentists has been provided by the Dental Sedation Teachers' Group (DSTG) in its document *The Competent Graduate*. Guidance for the training of dental nurses is provided by the National Examining Board for Dental Nurses. Both dentists and nurses should keep a log of their clinical experience (Figs 9-4 and 9-5).

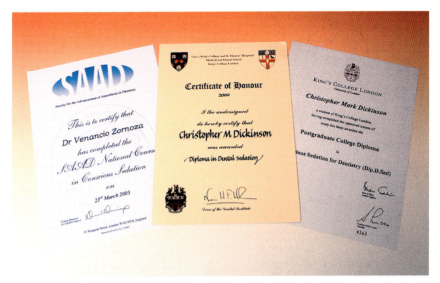

Fig 9-2 Certificates demonstrating evidence of conscious sedation training for dentists.

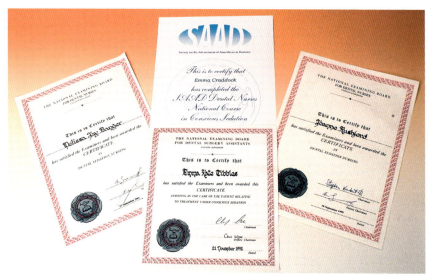

Fig 9-3 Certificates demonstrating evidence of conscious sedation training for nurses.

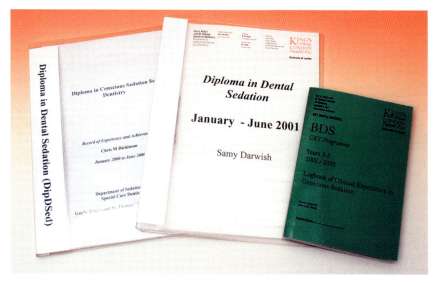

Fig 9-4 Postgraduate dentist's clinical log.

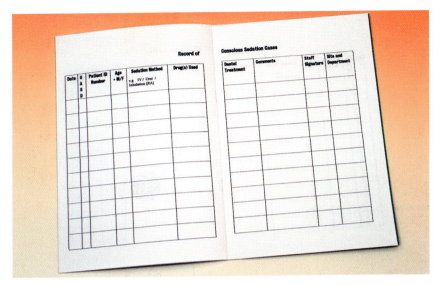

Fig 9-5 Dental nurse's clinical log.

Undergraduate education and training

The undergraduate course presents a unique opportunity to ensure that all dental graduates are able to provide safe conscious sedation for patients who find dentistry distressing. The GDC's framework for undergraduate dental education (*The First Five Years*) states that the control of anxiety and pain is fundamental to the practice of dentistry and that dental graduates must have had clinical experience in the administration of both inhalation and intravenous conscious sedation. This statement should not be taken to mean that all dental students are competent sedationists on graduation because, unfortunately, not all UK dental schools are currently able to provide sufficient clinical training. New dental graduates should, therefore, recognise their limited experience in the use of conscious sedation and undertake supplementary postgraduate study as required.

The Dental Sedation Teachers' Group has suggested a standard of clinical experience which should enable the new graduate to provide unsupervised sedation for fit individuals needing uncomplicated dentistry. It is recommended that this minimum level of experience should be:

- 5 patient assessments.
- 10 inhalational sedation cases.
- 20 intravenous sedation cases.

Postgraduate education and training

There are a number of options open to dentists seeking postgraduate training in conscious sedation. These include:

- short courses (1–3 days)
- clinical experience programmes
- diploma courses
- master's degrees.

Short courses are offered by the postgraduate dental deaneries, by dental teaching hospitals and private organisations – for example the Society for the Advancement of Anaesthesia in Dentistry (SAAD). These usually provide good theoretical instruction and skills practice but cannot offer clinical training and hands-on experience with patients. Such experience has to be sought on an individual basis on completion of a short course. At present there is no formal mechanism for this apart from small-scale mentoring schemes such as those offered by DSTG and SAAD. The Department of Health has recognised the difficulty of accessing clinical experience and has devised a National Course in Conscious Sedation (England and Wales). Sadly, this initiative has not been supported by sufficient funding.

Short programmes of clinical experience are sometimes offered by regional maxillofacial units and some dental teaching hospital departments. The experience available may be limited to particular groups of patients and sedation techniques.

Diplomas are offered by a few UK dental schools (e.g. Guy's, King's and St Thomas' (GKT) Dental Institute, King's College, London; Newcastle-upon-Tyne). These diplomas are awarded by the university dental hospitals following the successful completion of a formal academic programme and assessment. The diploma programmes, which extend over 9 to 12 months (1,200 hours of study), typically include:

- formal teaching sessions (lectures, seminars)
- extensive hands-on clinical practice
- self-directed learning
- continuous assessment (tutor-marked essays, MCQs)
- workplace audit
- written, clinical and oral examinations
- dissertation.

Some university dental hospitals also offer a shorter (600 hours) postgraduate certificate in conscious sedation. At the time of writing there is only one

UK Master's degree programme, offered by the GKT Dental Institute, which includes a substantial sedation component. This is a two-year, full-time academic programme in sedation and special care dentistry intended for dentists wishing to pursue a career in these areas of practice.

Retention and improvement of knowledge and skills rely upon regular updating by means of appropriate refresher courses. The intervals after which updating is required will depend upon individual circumstances but should be documented.

Environment and Equipment for Sedation

The treatment and recovery areas must be of sufficient size to allow adequate access for the patient, the dental team and the sedation equipment. The dental chair and recovery trolley/chair must be capable of being placed in the head-down tilt position.

Inhalational sedation
- A purpose-designed, regularly maintained Relative Analgesia machine must be used.
- Non-interchangeable, colour-coded pipelines must be used.
- Failsafe mechanisms must be in place to ensure that hypoxic mixtures cannot be delivered.
- Gas cylinders must be stored safely according to current regulations.
- Scavenging of waste gases must conform to current COSHH standards.
- Nasal masks (without air entrainment valves) should provide a good seal.

Intravenous sedation
- All the appropriate intravenous and monitoring equipment must be available in the treatment area.
- Supplemental oxygen and intermittent positive pressure ventilation equipment must be immediately available.
- Calibrated and appropriately maintained equipment is required for all infusion techniques.

Indications for Conscious Sedation
- To treat anxious or phobic patients who are unlikely otherwise to accept treatment.
- To enable unpleasant procedures to be carried out without distress.
- To avoid general anaesthesia.

Patient selection

Careful assessment of the patient ensures that correct decisions are made regarding treatment planning. The simplest technique which is likely to be successful should be chosen in the first instance. This technique is selected taking into consideration the patient's age, state of health, social circumstances and any special needs or contraindications to specific drugs.

Remember that only patients in ASA categories I and II should be treated outside specialist centres. The clinical environment and the skills of the sedation team must also be considered. Treatment under sedation should only proceed if the sedationist is satisfied that all these criteria can be met.

Patient preparation

All patients who are to receive treatment under conscious sedation must be given clear verbal and written instructions. Fasting is not normally required. Patients should be advised to take only light food and clear non–alcoholic fluids prior to the appointment. A responsible adult escort must be available to accompany the patient home (or to a suitable place of care) and to assume responsibility during the post-sedation period.

In the case of intravenous and oral sedation techniques, the patient should be supervised for the remainder of the day. This may mean that outpatient conscious sedation cannot be offered for an individual who lives alone or who is the sole carer for children, elderly or dependent relatives. In situations where an adult patient has been sedated by nitrous oxide and oxygen only, prolonged supervision is usually unnecessary.

Wherever possible, the patient and escort should travel home by private car or taxi rather than public transport. If this cannot be arranged, the escort must be made aware of the added responsibilities of caring for the patient during the journey home. If either the patient or their escort appears unwilling to comply with these requirements, conscious sedation should not be offered.

Consent

Specific written consent must be obtained from all patients who are to receive treatment under sedation. The principles set out in *A Reference Guide to Consent for Examination or Treatment*, published by the Department of Health, must be followed.

Written consent must be obtained in advance of the procedure (the assessment visit offers a suitable opportunity). It is important to remember that the mere presence of a signature does not guarantee that the consent obtained is valid. For consent to be valid it must be given voluntarily by an appropriately informed person (the patient or someone with parental responsibility for a patient under 16 years of age). Mere acquiescence, where the person does not know or is unable to understand what the intervention entails, does NOT constitute valid consent. The process of consent to treatment is an ever-changing area of clinical practice. It is therefore important to keep up to date with developments.

Patients who are already sedated cannot, under any circumstances, be regarded as competent to take decisions regarding consent for treatment. It is therefore highly unsatisfactory to seek consent for dental treatment from a sedated patient.

All decisions made by patients in respect of their treatment must be based on sound information and personal choice. The dentist should present options for pain and anxiety control and professional advice. Patients should not be coerced to accept any form of treatment if they do not wish to do so by members of the dental team or relatives or friends, no matter how well meaning their intentions. If a treatment plan cannot be predetermined (perhaps because of extreme anxiety relating to even a dental examination), an explanation, in broad terms, of the possible treatment options should be given and agreed.

Clinical Records and Procedures

Accurate clinical records are essential for every patient. The following information should be recorded for all patients undergoing treatment under conscious sedation:
- A full medical, dental and social history, including prescribed and self-prescribed medication, alcohol consumption, tobacco habits and drug abuse.
- Previous conscious sedation/general anaesthetic history.
- Presedation assessment, including any individual patient requirements.
- Written instructions provided.
- Availability of suitable escort and aftercare.
- Compliance with the pretreatment instructions.
- Written consent obtained for conscious sedation and dental treatment.
- Any changes in the recorded medical or drug history.
- Monitoring – clinical and electronic.
- Dose, route and times of administration of sedation agents, including any problems.

- Dental treatment details, including plan for next visit.
- Post-sedation assessment and time of discharge.

Aftercare

Recovery from sedation is a progressive process. The initial phase usually takes place in the dental chair and is supervised directly by the dentist or the "second appropriate person". Patients may later be moved to a suitably equipped and staffed recovery area or a waiting room where they can be reunited with their escort. Drowsy patients should not be transferred to a public area: this is often embarrassing for the individual who has received sedation and for other patients waiting to be seen.

The decision to discharge a patient into the care of an escort following any type of sedation must be the responsibility of the sedationist. The patient MUST be able to walk unaided, without stumbling or feeling unstable, before being allowed to leave professional supervision. Adult patients who have received nitrous oxide and oxygen inhalation sedation alone may leave unaccompanied at the discretion of the dentist.

Medicolegal Requirements for Specific Sedation Techniques and Circumstances

Inhalation sedation

The only currently recommended technique for inhalation sedation is the use of a titrated dose of nitrous oxide with oxygen. It is absolutely essential that safeguards are in place to ensure that a hypoxic mixture cannot be administered. During inhalation sedation, clinical monitoring of the patient without additional electromechanical devices is generally adequate.

Intravenous sedation

The generally agreed standard technique for intravenous sedation is the use of a titrated dose of a single benzodiazepine. Continuous propofol infusion has gained some popularity in recent years and other drugs or combinations of drugs may be appropriate in specially selected circumstances. It is emphasised their use must be restricted to a fully trained and experienced practitioner working in specialist practice.

All syringes must be clearly labelled so that those containing dental materials, local anaesthetics and sedative drugs can be readily identified (Fig 9-6). This is particularly important where a number of syringes are loaded, where

122

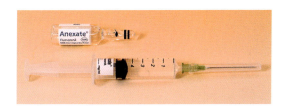

Fig 9-6 Labelled syringe.

containers have labels of a similar colour and layout or where a drug is available in a number of concentrations. Each drug should be given according to accepted recommendations for administration and titration.

The use of fixed doses or bolus techniques is unacceptable in both inhalation and intravenous conscious sedation as safety is directly related to titration of the dose according to the individual patient's needs.

All members of the clinical team must be capable of monitoring the condition of the patient. For intravenous sedation, continuous pulse oximetry is mandatory.

Oral and intranasal sedation
Oral premedication with a low dose of a sedative agent may be prescribed to assist with sleep the night before, or to reduce anxiety on the day of treatment. This must be clearly differentiated from oral and intranasal techniques of sedation which require special training and experience and should only be used in specialist practice. Special consent must be obtained for sedatives not currently licensed for these applications.

Conscious Sedation for Children

Conscious sedation must be undertaken only by teams which have adequate training and experience in case selection, behavioural management and administration of sedation for children and only in an appropriate environment.

Nitrous oxide and oxygen should be the first choice for paediatric dental patients who are unable to tolerate treatment with local anaesthesia alone and who have a sufficient level of understanding to accept the procedure. Intravenous, oral and intranasal sedation techniques are rarely necessary for children and must only be provided by those who are trained and experienced in these paediatric sedation techniques.

Complications

The management of any complication requires the **whole** dental team to be:

- aware of the risk of complications
- trained in basic life support
- trained and regularly rehearsed in emergency procedures
- equipped with appropriate means of airway protection and oxygen delivery
- able to use emergency drugs
- aware of the need to keep adequate supplies of in-date emergency drugs and oxygen.

Clinical Governance and Audit

It is a requirement of good practice that all clinicians work with colleagues to monitor and maintain awareness of the quality of the care that they provide for their patients. This is a basic principle of clinical governance and risk management. Attention must be given to risk awareness, risk control, risk containment and risk transfer. Evidence of active participation in continuing professional education and personal clinical audit is an essential feature of clinical governance.

Conclusions

- The practice of conscious sedation is strictly regulated in the UK.
- Opportunities for undergraduate and postgraduate training have increased but are still limited.

Further Reading

Department of Health. A Reference Guide to Consent for Examination or Treatment. London: HMSO, 2001.

General Dental Council. Maintaining Standards. London: GDC, 2001.

Index

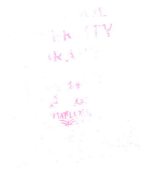

Quintessentials for General Dental Practitioners Series

in 36 volumes

Editor-in-Chief: Professor Nairn H F Wilson

The Quintessentials for General Dental Practitioners Series covers basic principles and key issues in all aspects of modern dental medicine. Each book can be read as a stand-alone volume or in conjunction with other books in the series.

Publication date, approximately

Oral Surgery and Oral Medicine, Editor: John G Meechan

Practical Dental Local Anaesthesia	available
Practical Oral Medicine	Spring 2004
Practical Conscious Sedation	available
Practical Surgical Dentistry	Spring 2004

Imaging, Editor: Keith Horner

Interpreting Dental Radiographs	available
Panoramic Radiology	Spring 2004
Twenty-first Century Dental Imaging	Autumn 2004

Periodontology, Editor: Iain L C Chapple

Understanding Periodontal Diseases: Assessment and Diagnostic Procedures in Practice	available
Decision-Making for the Periodontal Team	available
Successful Periodontal Therapy – A Non-Surgical Approach	available
Periodontal Management of Children, Adolescents and Young Adults	available
Periodontal Medicine: A Window on the Body	Spring 2004

Implantology, Editor: Lloyd J Searson

Implantology in General Dental Practice	Spring 2004
Managing Orofacial Pain in Practice	Spring 2004

Endodontics, Editor: John M Whitworth

Rational Root Canal Treatment in Practice	available
Managing Endodontic Failure in Practice	Spring 2004
Managing Dental Trauma in Practice	Spring 2004
Preventing Pulpal Injury in Practice	Autumn 2005

Prosthodontics, Editor: P Finbarr Allen

Teeth for Life for Older Adults	available
Complete Dentures – from Planning to Problem Solving	available
Removable Partial Dentures – A Systematic Approach	Spring 2004
Fixed Prosthodontics for the General Dental Practitioner	Autumn 2005
Occlusion: A Theoretical and Team Approach	Autumn 2004

Operative Dentistry, Editor: Paul A Brunton

Decision-Making in Operative Dentistry	available
Applied Dental Materials in Operative Dentistry	Spring 2005
Aesthetic Dentistry	Spring 2004
Indirect Restorations	Autumn 2004
Psychological and Behavioural Management of Adult Dental Patients	Autumn 2004

Paediatric Dentistry/Orthodontics, Editor: Marie Therese Hosey

Child Taming: How to Cope with Children in Dental Practice	available
Paediatric Cariology	Spring 2004
Treatment Planning for the Developing Dentition	Autumn 2004

General Dentistry and Practice Management, Editor: Raj Rattan

The Business of Dentistry	available
Risk Management	Spring 2004
Practice Management for the Dental Team	Autumn 2004
IT in Dentistry: A Working Manual	Autumn 2005
Quality Assurance	Autumn 2004
Dental Practice Design	Spring 2005

Quintessence Publishing Co. Ltd., London